PUBLIC HEALTH IN THE 21ST CENTURY

ACCIDENTAL FALLS

RISK FACTORS, PREVENTION STRATEGIES AND LONG-TERM OUTCOMES

PUBLIC HEALTH IN THE 21ST CENTURY

Additional books in this series can be found on Nova's website under the Series tab.

Additional e-books in this series can be found on Nova's website under the e-book tab.

PUBLIC HEALTH IN THE 21ST CENTURY

ACCIDENTAL FALLS

RISK FACTORS, PREVENTION STRATEGIES AND LONG-TERM OUTCOMES

BRENDA EVANS
EDITOR

nova publishers
New York

NOTICE TO THE READER

Library of Congress Cataloging-in-Publication Data

ISBN: 978-1-63483-228-1

Published by Nova Science Publishers, Inc. † New York

CONTENTS

PREFACE

Falls are considered as one of the accidents that take more loss of functionality, mainly in older adults. This book begins with a discussion on the prevalence of falls among different populations, the most used definitions and classifications for falls and their physical, social and psychological consequences. Furthermore, this book provides easy and practical recommendations for falls and fall-related injury prevention.

Chapter 1 - Falls are considered as one of the accidents that take more loss of functionality, mainly in older adults. This chapter describes the prevalence of falls among different populations, the most used definitions and classifications for falls and their physical, social and psychological consequences. Health professional and society need to know the main risk factors for falls in order to screen older adults at greater risk and draw correct prevention strategies. The authors talked about the importance of identifying the combination of risk factors presented in each person. Since the prevalence of falls increases to 60% among older people with cognitive impairment and their consequences tend to be more serious, a brief text was inserted in this chapter. A large amount of sensitive methods has been described to assess falls and screen susceptible people for this event. This chapter helps health professionals to select the most appropriate tools to each patient or target population. Finally, prevention and rehabilitation strategies were mentioned, thinking about the complex interaction between environment, individual and task. To reduce the public health burden and fall-related injuries, it is imperative that effective preventive strategies are put in place.

Chapter 2 - This work aims to provide easy and practical recommendations for falls and fall-related injuries prevention set on the analysis of a theoretical dynamic system involving the subject (older adult), the environment, and the task performance.

In accordance with this system, accidental falls occur while performing physical activities/tasks. In the absence of movement the probability of falling will be almost zero. However, immobility decreases the subject´s ability of performance. The fall usually occurs when the demands of a given task exceed the subject's ability. The demands of a task are determined by its difficulty and by environmental conditions. In a hostile environment, the demands of a given task increase. As result, the task demands may exceed the subject's ability causing a fall.

The ability to perform daily tasks without falling tends to decline with age due to associated frailty (notably the increased morbidities and the diminished physical, sensorial, and neural fitness). However, falls may also be a problem before the age of 60 years. The main immediate consequence of a fall is injury, which may be fatal. Another possible short-term consequence is an increased fear of falling that often conducts to a loss of independence while performing daily tasks and, consequently, leads to a decline in the subject's ability.

It was observed that the determinant factor for the rupture of this system balance (resulting in falls and fall-related injuries) in older adults is the subject, namely his/her condition of frailty. As the subject becomes more fragile and as the risk of intrinsic factors increases, their susceptibility to extrinsic factors rises, especially with regard to environmental hazards. Thereafter, the subject's likelihood of falling and injuring increases. However, a good level of physical fitness can also increase the threat of falling and injuring, because fitter people are more confidence in performing more demanding tasks and in more hazardous environments. Thereby, they expose themselves to more dangerous situations.

Given the above and reporting recent research findings, the primary recommendations for fall and fall-related injuries prevention are the following:

- A healthy lifestyle, in order to avoid co-morbidities or, at least, to minimize its effects.
- The reduction of environmental hazards, principally when fitness decreases and frailty increases, and the restraint of difficult tasks in hazardous environments.
- The practice at least 1,150 MET-min.wk^{-1} of physical activity, with no more than 500 MET-min.wk^{-1} (~60 min. wk^{-1}) of vigorous physical activity (due to associated hazards). For example a combination of 1 hour of walking, 2 hours of moderate physical activity (such as

carrying light loads or bicycling at a regular pace) and 20 minutes of vigorous physical activity (such as heavy lifting, digging, aerobics, or fast bicycling) per week, what computes ~1,150 MET-min.wk^{-1}.

- The implementation of exercise programs to prevent physical fitness loss, especially balance. Further, muscle strength and gait exercises may be particularly relevant for less fit and frail people.
- The performance of functional exercises that mimic everyday life tasks and promote self-confidence.
- Regarding women, special attention must be taken because they tend to be more fragile. Regarding men, special attention must be taken because they tend to expose themselves to more hazardous situations.

Chapter 3 - A sensorimotor approach that included the use of repetitive, fast, and gross movement patterns was chosen for as the theoretical foundation for this case study. This approach is intended for use across disciplines and the principles of this approach have been correlated with fall prevention in persons who have a diagnosis of Parkinson's disease. It was hypothesized that there would be a significant decrease in the reported number of falls following successful completion of intervention that consisted of the use of the sensorimotor approach to intervention. The intervention included preparatory, purposeful, and occupation-based interventions using fast, repetitive gross motor patterns of movement. The goal of this sensorimotor approach was to teach the participant a new way of moving that would now be required in order to safety engage in everyday occupations. The process of learning and using new ways of moving by altering the effort required and type of movement required for task completion is a phenomenon referred to in the literature as "recalibration." Upon completion of the intervention, the participant had achieved success in gaining a new awareness of the effort required to internally regulate the movements required for safe and successful completion of occupations of daily living. The average rate of reported falls prior to the participant's participation in the study was one per month and at six month follow-up from the initiation of his participation in the study, patient had no falls to report.

Chapter 4 - In Brazil and in the United States, the prevalence of falls is approximately 30%. A lot of measures have been adopted trying to reduce this rate; however, the number of older adults who fall is still rising. Falling is associated with increased disability rates, as well as hospital and nursing home admissions. Research has identified many risk factors for falling, including physical and environmental hazards. In addition, as many chronic diseases older adults present, higher is the risk of falling. Self-perceived health has been used in research as a good indicator of individuals' actual health. Using a secondary dataset the relationship between self-perceived health and falls was tested in community dwelling older adults from the state of Rio Grande do Sul, Brazil. The data were used to test whether self-perceived health is associated with falling, controlling for sociodemographic variables (age, gender and monthly household income). Analysis was conducted using bivariate cross tabulation and noting of chi-square values. To sum up, self-perceived health has a relationship with falls and this is an important finding since inquiring self-perceived health is a simple and fast measure that might be useful in identifying older adults at risk of falling.

Chapter 5 - Increasing traction properties of the floor surface would be desirable as a general rule, but a very high level of slip-resistance may impede safe and comfortable ambulation. There is lack of evidences whether traction properties are linearly correlated with surface features of the floor or what levels of floor surface finishes are required to effective control of slipperiness. It is also scarce to find studies and/or guidelines on the operational ranges of floor surface roughness required for optimal slip-resistance performance. The objectives of this chapter are to investigate the effects of floor surface finishes on slip-resistance performance under different environmental and shoe-type conditions, and identify operational ranges of floor surface roughness as practical design information for the prevention of fall incidents. A theory model of three operative zones was suggested to characterize functional levels of floor surface roughness on slip-resistance performance. To test the theory model, dynamic friction tests were conducted using 3 shoes and 9 floor specimens under 2 lubricated environments: wet and soapy conditions. The test results showed that significant effects of floor-type on dynamic friction coefficient (DFC) were found in both lubricated conditions. As compared to the floor-type effects, shoe-type effects were relatively small. Slip-resistance performance was significantly affected by and well correlated with the floor surface roughness under the soapy environment. Polynomial regression analyses amongst the floor surface roughness, DFCs and environments allowed to estimating operational ranges for optimal slip-resistance performance. Under the soapy environment, floor surfaces with 17 and 52 μm in *Ra* roughness parameter most likely represented the lower and upper bounds of the operational ranges. The test result also identified that the soapsuds-covered soapy floors required rougher surface finishes than the wet ones in their lower boundary roughness range. However, there were lack of correlations between the surface roughness and slip-resistance properties under the wet surface condition. The current study suggests that designs for the floor surface finishes would require different levels of surface roughness for different types of environmental conditions to effectively control slippery walking environments.

Chapter 6 - Pedestrian falls resulting from slips and/or trips are one of the leading categories of non-traffic incidents in terms of serious injuries and fatalities. They are a primary cause of industry injuries, as well as one of the leading causes of injury-related deaths for the elderly aged 65 and over. Fall incidents involve multi-factors, but have been commonly assessed by slip-resistance measurements as a simplified format of coefficient of friction (COF) quantity amongst shoes, floors and environments. However, slip-resistance properties have unique and specific features to any combination of the shoe, floor and environment. Notwithstanding such complex characteristics, COFs consistently change because slip-resistance properties are inherently noisy and geometric dimensions between the shoes and floors are largely modified during repetitive measurements. Whilst controversies on the friction measurements for the evaluation of slipperiness remain, slip-resistance properties are still commonly measured by COF readings in many studies and practices for slip and fall safety assessments. To enhance the validity and reliability of friction measurements, therefore, it is necessary to improve our understanding on the slip-resistance mechanics, mechanisms, and related tribo-physical characteristics of the sliding interface amongst the shoes, floors and environments. Because surface topographies of the shoes and floors are largely modified throughout the course of ambulation, this may considerably affect friction and wear behaviours and be one of the most important factors on the slip-resistance properties. Furthermore, surface features significantly affect the degree of slip-resistance performance and have a direct correlation to the ease of cleaning. A high profile surface finish is hard to clean and eventually loses its texture due to inability to remove dirt and physical erosions of the floor surface. This will also increase the risk of slipperiness. However, these issues are hardly investigated in the literature. This study explores the current knowledge gaps and misinterpretations on slip-resistance measurements that are mainly caused by oversimplified perceptions on friction phenomena between the shoes and floors and suggests a new paradigm on slip-resistance assessments for future researches on pedestrian fall incidents.

In: Accidental Falls
Editor: Brenda Evans

ISBN: 978-1-63483-228-1

Chapter 1

FALLS IN OLDER PEOPLE: PREVALENCE, RISK FACTORS, ASSESSMENT AND INTERVENTION STRATEGIES

Juliana Hotta Ansai, Thais Rabiatti Aurichio and Larissa Pires de Andrade

[1]Postgraduate Program of Physiotherapy, Federal University of São Carlos, São Carlos, Brazil

[2]Postgraduate Program of Physiotherapy, Federal University of São Carlos, São Carlos, Brazil

[3]Physiotherapy Department, Federal University of São Carlos, São Carlos, Brazil

ABSTRACT

Falls are considered as one of the accidents that take more loss of functionality, mainly in older adults. This chapter describes the prevalence of falls among different populations, the most used definitions and classifications for falls and their physical, social and psychological consequences. Health professional and society need to know the main risk factors for falls in order to screen older adults at greater risk and draw correct prevention strategies. The authors talked about the importance of identifying the combination of risk factors presented in each person. Since the prevalence of falls increases to 60% among older people with cognitive impairment and their consequences tend to be more serious, a brief text was inserted in this chapter. A large amount of sensitive methods has been described to assess falls and screen susceptible people for this event. This chapter helps health professionals to select the most appropriate tools to each patient or target population. Finally, prevention and rehabilitation strategies were mentioned, thinking about the complex interaction between environment, individual and task. To reduce the public health burden and fall-related injuries, it is imperative that effective preventive strategies are put in place.

Keywords: Falls, fall-related injuries, risk factors, assessment, prevention

INTRODUCTION

According to World Health Organization (2008), the global elderly population is increasing dramatically. In 2006, the number of people over 60 was 650 million. By 2050, it is expected to reach two billion people and 80% of them will be found in developing countries. Although more people are keeping their good health along the years, aging still increases risk of physical and functional frailty and loss of autonomy and quality of life (Rubenstein, 2006).

One of the accidents that take more loss of functionality is falls. This event is considered as one of the geriatric giants. Falls occur at any age and even in healthy people. However, the concern is not only related to the high incidence of falls in older people, but rather the combination of high incidence and susceptibility to injury (Rubenstein, 2006; Peel, 2011).

The rate of falls among older adults varies widely in the literature, due to differences in study population characteristics, methods of falls data ascertainment and reporting. According to Liu-Ambrose et al. (2008), approximately 30% of community-dwelling older adults fall one or more times each year. Among adults aged 80 years old and over, this rate reaches 50% (Anderson, 2008). However, in China, the overall median annual incidence was 18%. The possible reasons for this lower incidence of falls are related to ethnicity, health, behavioral and lifestyle factors (Kwan et al., 2011). Moreover, 64% of falls occur in the bathroom, 66% occur during the night and 77% are not assisted (Clyburn & Heydemann, 2011). In 75% of cases, people are walking, sitting or getting up (Perracini & Ramos, 2002).

Among older people with cognitive impairment, the prevalence of falls increases to 60% and their consequences tend to be more serious (Liu-Ambrose et al., 2008). In adults between 75 and 84 years old who need help in activities of daily living, the probability to fall is 14 times higher than in independent people with the same age (Perracini, 2005). The rate of falls may also vary according to the study site. Because of a high prevalence of chronic diseases, functional disability and age-related physiological changes, older people in care settings are more vulnerable to falls and fall-related injury (Rubenstein, 2006). In acute care settings, falls accounted for 30 to 40% of reported safety incidents (Oliver & Healy, 2009). Residents have an incidence of falls nearly five times more than community dwelling people of the same age (Australian Commission on Safety and Quality in Health Care, 2009).

Although at first what is fall seems to be obvious, health professionals and researchers can interpret a fall in different ways. Therefore, the adoption of a standardized definition is necessary for consistency and comparison of outcome measures. One of the most used definitions of falls is "an event which results in a person coming to rest inadvertently on the ground or floor or other lower level and other than as a consequence of the following: sustaining a violent blow; loss of consciousness; sudden onset of paralysis; or an epileptic seizure" (Chiu; Au-Yeung & Lo, 2003). For purposes in injury surveillance systems, accidental falls may be classified as falls on the same level (e.g., slipping or tripping) or on different levels (e.g., stairs, ladder, bed or other structure) (Peel, 2011).

Regarding number of falls within six months, falls can be classified as occasional (one fall in one year) and recurrent (two or more) (Stel et al., 2003). A quarter to half of fallers experienced recurrent falls, with higher rates of recurrent falls (75%) in older people over 85 years old (Fleming et al., 2008). Furthermore, more than two thirds of people who suffer a fall will fall again within the subsequent six months (Perracini, 2005). Occasional falls are caused mainly by extrinsic factors (i.e., environmental factors), whereas recurrent falls are usually caused by intrinsic factors (i.e., physical, cognitive and behavioral factors within the person) (Stel et al., 2003). These factors are better explained at RISK FACTORS section.

As mentioned before, the problem is the high incidence and consequences related to falls (Rubenstein, 2006; Peel, 2011). Falls can lead to physical, social and psychological consequences, contributing to restricted activities, early homebound status, reduced mobility and dependence (Rubenstein, 2006). In prospective studies, 60 to 75% of falls provided injuries, most of which were minor (swollen joints, bruises, abrasions) (Kwan et al., 2011). Although most falls do not produce serious injury, 10 to 15% produce serious injuries, such as fractures, joint dislocations and head injuries (Peel, 2011). In hospitals, 30% of all falls lead to injury and 1 to 5% lead to serious injury (Healey et al., 2008).

Among all injuries related to falls, fractures provide the largest health care burden. Approximately 5 to 10% of falls result in a fracture. Furthermore, 90% of all fractures are attributable to falls (Peeters & Lips, 2009). Luukinen et al. (1997) verified that fear of falling, decreased muscle strength, high social participation and poor distance vision increased the risk of a fall-related fracture. Among older people, fall-related fractures are more often during slips, trips and falls due to extrinsic factors such as being pulled or collisions (Luukinen et al., 2000).

One of the most known psychological consequences is the post-fall anxiety syndrome or fear of falling. Fear of falling can cause an older person to restrict its activities, lose confidence in the ability to ambulate safely and ambulate less frequently. Consequently, this person can present weakness and reduced balance, functional decline, depression and social isolation, resulting in decreased quality of life and autonomy and increased risk of falling (Rubenstein, 2006; Pell, 2011).

Furthermore, falls result in increased social and health care costs (Anderson, 2008; Chang et al., 2004). According to World Health Organization (2007), costs related to fall can be categorized into two aspects: direct and indirect costs. Direct costs involves health care costs such as medications, consultations in treatment and rehabilitation. Indirect costs are societal productivity losses of activities for individuals and family caregivers.

Falls correspond to the main reasons of high mortality and morbidity rates in older adults. Two third of deaths from accidents in older adults are attributable to falls (Rubenstein, 2006). Other consequences include inability to get up from the floor after falling, caregiver stress (National Ageing Research Institute, 2004), nursing home admission (Peel, 2011) and hospitalization. Only 50% of older adults admitted to hospital due to a fall recover their functional status after one year (Rubenstein, 2006).

Falls are a multifactorial and complex event. Identifying individuals with greater risk of falling is a major task and a large amount of sensitive methods has been described to assess falls and screen these susceptible people. To reduce the public health burden and fall-related injuries, it is imperative that effective preventive strategies are put in place.

RISK FACTORS

Identifying the profile of the most vulnerable older people to fall is important, as well as differing which of them have greater susceptibility to serious injuries caused by falls or are predisposed to suffer recurrent falls (Perracini, 2005). It is essential to determine the risk factors for falls in order to screen older adults at greater risk and draw correct prevention and rehabilitation strategies.

We can divide the risk factors for falls into intrinsic and extrinsic factors. Intrinsic factors refer to those that are inherent to the individual, such as muscle weakness, age and visual impairment. Extrinsic factors are determined by the environment or external conditions, such as low luminosity, polypharmacy and use of slipper shoes. Among older people under 75 years old, falls are more related to extrinsic factors, while intrinsic factors are more related to people aged 80 and older (Peel, 2011).

Intrinsic and extrinsic risk factors are also named as predisposing factors, since they lead to a greater chance to suffer falls. In contrast, causal factors are present in the occurrence of a specific event of fall and are the reasons that led the person to fall (Perracini, 2005). The causes of falls are closely related to the functional level of the older person and its performed tasks. It is very common to observe falls associated with poorly maintained sidewalks among active community-dwelling older adults. In contrast, institutionalized and hospitalized older people are more likely to fall from bed or during transfers. Elderly in rehabilitation are at increased risk of falls, with serious injuries, compared to those who are not in a rehabilitation process (Peel, 2011).

Accident and environment-related, gait, balance disorders or weakness, dizziness, drop attack, confusion, postural hypotension, visual disorder, syncope, other specified causes (arthritis, acute illness, drugs, alcohol, pain, epilepsy and falling from bed) and unknown variables were the most probable causes of falls mentioned by 12 retrospectives studies. However, the etiology of falls in elderly is multifactorial, which makes the selection of a single cause unviable. Furthermore, most older people present several determinable risk factors and identify them is much more useful than trying to classify specific precipitating causes retrospectively (Rubenstein, 2006).

Several studies have discussed risk factors for falls in elderly. Rubenstein (2006) analyzed 16 controlled studies and listed the main risk factors for falls in elderly. In order of importance, they are: muscle weakness, balance disorders, walking difficulties, visual impairment, mobility limitation, cognitive disorders, functional loss and hypotension postural. Evans et al. (2001), in a systematic review, studied risk factors in hospitals. They included 18 studies, which appointed impaired mental status, special toileting needs, impaired mobility, and a history of falling as factors associated with an increased risk of falling. The authors suggest that medications and advanced age can also influence a patient's risk of falling.

Perracini (2005) classified risk factors among elderly according to the frequency of their appearance in studies (High Risk for a factor presented in most studies; Medium Risk for a factor presented in a good part of the studies; and Low Risk for a factor presented in just one or two studies). These risk factors were also associated with occasional, recurrent falls or falls with serious injuries. Although the factors analyzed were not homogeneous, this classification serves as a guide to value risk factors with greater or lesser intensity (Table 1).

Table 1. Classification of risk factors for falls according to evidence and type of injury

HIGH RISK	MEDIUM RISK	LOW RISK
Female gender/Age≥75 years (occasional, recurrent and with injuries)	Visual impairment (occasional, recurrent and with injuries)	Cognitive impairment (occasional and recurrent)
Difficulty in daily living activities/Sedentarism and inactivity (occasional, recurrent and with injuries)	Urinary incontinence/Urge incontinence (recurrent and with injuries)	Living alone (with injuries)
Balance, gait or mobility disorders (occasional, recurrent and with injuries)	Dizziness complaint (occasional and recurrent)	Neuropathy (with injuries)
Previous falls and fractures (recurrent and with injuries)		Postural hypotension (recurrent)
Polypharmacy/use of psychotropic (recurrent and with injuries)		Absence of spouse/Fear of falling (recurrent)
Cognitive decline/Previous stroke (occasional and recurrent)		Previous hospitalization/Depression (occasional)
Muscle weakness of lower limbs (occasional and recurrent)		Need for walking aids, decreased reflexes and foot problems (occasional)

Adapted from Perracini (2005).

Some authors have attributed the use of inappropriate footwear as a risk factor for falls in elderly (Koepsell et al., 2004; Menant et al., 2008). The material of sole and its design can change the friction coefficient on different surfaces, which allows an older person to slip. The height and width of heel influence in gait and posture, while the thickness of sole and the heel support can alter proprioception (Koepsell et al., 2004).

Among community dwelling older people, the use of heels higher than 2.5 cm is strongly associated with falls (Tencer et al., 2004). Koepsell et al. (2004) found that walking barefoot or with socks increased risk of falls, compared to the use of athletic or canvas shoes. Kelsey et al. (2010) found that most of elderly who fell at home walked barefoot or wore slippers or socks.

A meta-analysis study conducted by Stubbs et al. (2014) concluded that chronic pain and feet pain are important risk factors for falls. Also, community older people with pain complaint were more likely to suffer falls in the previous year and to fall again in the future.

Tinetti et al. (1998) investigated mental, physical and household risk factors for falls in community older adults aging over 75 years. After one year of the study, the risk of falls linearly grew up to 8% in older people who had no risk factors for falls and to 78% in people who had four or more risk factors. Nevitt et al. (1989) also found similar results, that is, the presence of only one risk factor increased by 10% the risk of falls, while the presence of four or more risk factors increased by 69% the risk of falls.

Since the etiology of falls is multifactorial and older people present diverse risk factors, identifying the combination of risk factors presented in each older person seems to be much more important than determining isolated risks. Also, identifying early this combination of factors is the key to implementation of more effective prevention strategies.

Falls in People with Cognitive Impairment

One reason for the increased quantity of falls among elderly people with cognitive impairment may be related to changes in frontal cognitive functions, specifically executive functions (Sheridan & Hausdorf, 2007). Executive functions involve control of attention, working memory and problem solving and are associated with impaired balance and gait in older adults, especially in dual task situations (Van Iersel et al., 2008; Montero-Odasso et al., 2012). Falls are three times more frequent in patients with Alzheimer's disease compared to non-demented elderly (Imamura et al., 2000).

Older people without cognitive impairment can use brain mechanisms and thus use one or more components of postural control changes to maintain balance (Franssen et al., 1999). Balance deficits associated with pathological processes may be related to hypoactivation of prefrontal association cortex, causing a cognitive-motor dyssynchrony (Siu et al., 2008) and favoring the occurrence of falls.

Some studies bring the pre-dementia stage, in other words the mild cognitive impairment. It may change gait kinematic parameters and precede the diagnosis of dementia (Hall et al., 2000; Verghese et al., 2007; Burachio et al., 2010). The early identification of dementia markers helps to identify patients at high risk of developing this condition. Consequently, it reflects the development of interventions that can mitigate occurrence of falls in this population.

In more advanced stages of cognitive impairment, such as Alzheimer's disease in moderate to severe stages, there may be presence of parkinsonian signs: akinesia, plastic rigidity, light tremor at rest, presence of some primitive reflexes (sucking, hold and glabellar) and hiperrelexia in deep tendon reflexes due to disinhibit motor and degenerative injury pre motor areas (Kato & Radanovic, 2008). These manifestations associated with cognitive impairment may further enhance the number of falls.

Given these motor and cognitive changes, it is necessary to deep assessments of measures of falls in older people with cognitive impairment, considering the high prevalence of falls in this population and their severe consequences.

How to Assess Falls and Screen People with Risk of Falls

Maintenance of balance depends on a complex interaction between environment, individual and task. Therefore, the assessment of falls in older people needs to approach different external conditions that may affect the responses to a stimulus, interaction of multiple sensory-motor processes, planning and execution of movements, presence of comorbidities and still the goal to be achieved in response to a stimulus.

In order to investigate the fall event, Perracini (2005) proposed a list of questions to approach elderly, such as: How many times did you fall in the last year? Was there any consequence? Was there a need to look for a doctor or an emergency service? Did you restrict your usual activities because of the fall? If so, was your restriction related to pain, insecurity, fear, difficult to walk? Talking about your last fall, when did it happen (day/night)? Did this event happen after a meal? Where did it happen? Were you conscious? What movements and activities were you doing at the time of the fall (walking, getting up, turning, bathing, wearing the slipper)? How did the fall happen (overbalance, distorted knees, weakness, dizzy)? What part of the body did you first hit on the floor or furniture? Were you wearing glasses or hearing aid (if applicable)? How were you in the previous week before falling? Was there any change in your medications? Did you think it is difficult to perform your daily activities?

Perracini (2005) also targeted action strategies after discriminating possible factors involved (Figure 1).

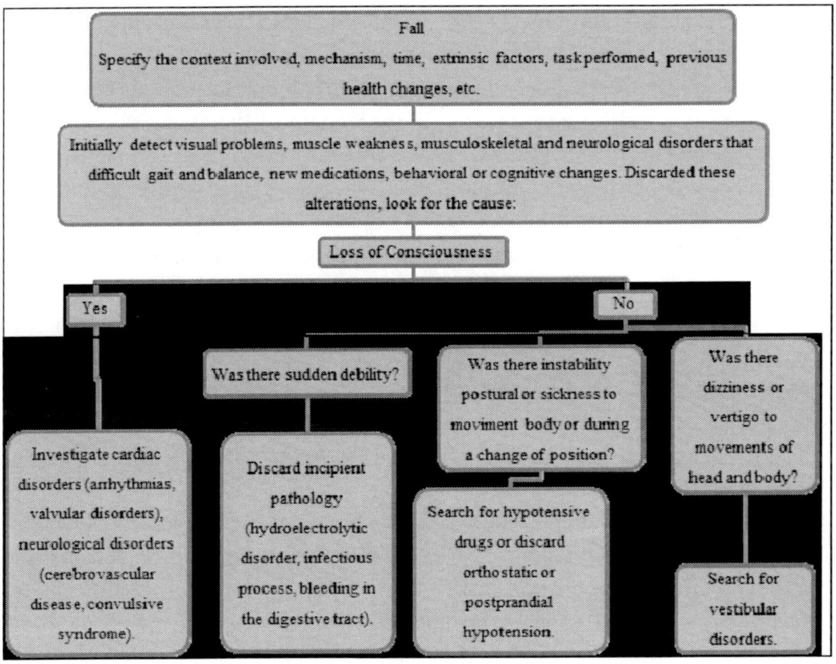

Figure 1. Algorithm to assess risk of falls in elderly (Perracini, 2005).

Based on the initial investigation, all aspects involved in the maintenance of balance need to be approached. Regarding the environment, it is extremely important to assess where the older person fell and the risks presented in this place. In order to detect early risk of falls, it is crucial to assess the person's home and the most frequented places. In outdoor environments, quality of pavement, tree roots apparent, irregular and poorly marked stairs, accessibility to public and commercial buildings (such as health centers, banks, pharmacies, markets), excess visual information, extremely busy environments and with difficult locomotion need to be observed.

In indoor environment, specifically at home, we need to identify carpets without fixation; slippery floors; poor lighting; furniture that is blocking passage; presence of pets or toys on the floor; irregular and not flagged steps; absence of handrails on stairs and grab bars in bathrooms; beds, chairs or couches with excessively low or high heights which can difficult transfers; and accessibility of common objects. In order to facilitate the assessment of older person's home, Rodriguez et al. (1995) proposed an environmental assessment tool to check risk of falls, named as Home Environment Survey (HES).

Shoes should also be assessed in the screening of risk of falls. Smooth or worn soles and flip flops should be discouraged. In contrast, anti-skid soles with excessive coefficient of friction to surface may cause stumbling and need to be avoided. The flexibility of sole is also an aspect to be considered. It should not be too rigid and prevent the propulsion of step, nor too flexible enough to be able to fold on forefoot and promote stumbling. Assess if the footwear used is appropriate to the foot length, its width and height are properly adjusted to foot dimensions and if the footwear is offering comfort, mobility and safety are the most important aspects to avoid injury, foot pain and falls in elderly. Therefore, footwear with good attachment to the foot, with adjustments such as laces and buckles and those that allow good handling of ankle should be advised.

Perhaps more important, another aspect involved in maintaining balance is the individual. The evaluation of the individual is based on motor, sensory and psychocognitive components involved in postural control. Among motor aspects, it is necessary to assess muscle strength, especially resistance and muscle power of lower limbs. The assessment of postural alignment and flexibility of lower limbs and spine can identify possible restrictions within limits of stability and low efficiency of adjustments in imbalance situations.

Balance and muscle strength of lower limbs in community elderly can be assessed through the Five Times Sit-to-Stand Test (FTSST). Initially, the person sits in a standard chair with 43 cm of height and without armrest. The person remains with arms crossed and it is instructed to get up until fully extend its knee and sit down for five times, as fast as it can. The timer stops when the person get up in the fifth repetition and the time spent is noted. Values over 14.2 s indicate balance disorders in community elderly (Whitney et al., 2005).

Regarding to sensory components, visual, vestibular and somatosensory (skin-protection sensitivity and joint proprioception) systems are an important part of the assessment of risk of falls. The organization and interaction of these three systems can be assessed by the Clinical Test of Sensory Interaction and Balance (CTSIB) (Shumway-Cook & Horak, 1986). This test provides information about individual's ability to adapt and maintain balance forward conditions of sensory conflict. Furthermore, it reveals which sensory system (visual, proprioceptive or vestibular) the person is more dependent to the maintenance of postural control (Perracini & Gazzola, 2011).

The assessment of psychocognitive components involves attentional aspects, such as performing motor tasks associated with cognitive tasks. These tests are called dual task tests and they can be used to screen risk of falls in elderly, since they represent everyday situations in which elderly need to perform tasks simultaneously. There is a competition for resources of central processing between postural control and other competitor tasks (cognitive or motor or motor-cognitive), which affects performance in both tasks and predisposes elderly to falls.

Fear of falling is another important psychocognitive aspect in the screening of risk of falls in older people, either people who have already suffered falls or those who never feel. Older people with fear of falling can present deterioration in balance control and avoid challenging situations, which restrict activities and predispose to inactivity, social isolation and other risk factors for new falls (Perracini, 2011). The Falls Efficacy Scale International (FES-I), described by Yardley et al. (2005), indicates how much the individual is concerned to fall in certain situations. Despite methodological particularities, the current literature scores 23 or more points as an elevated concern about falling (Delbaere et al., 2010).

Other important aspects in the individual assessment are anticipatory postural and reactive (ankle, hip and step strategies) responses to external disturbances (Unphred, 2004). Elderly tend to use the hip strategy even in small displacements, in which the ankle strategy would be preferred. They tend to use step strategy (considered as protective reaction) in low challenging situations, which points deficit in postural control. Such strategies may be evaluated alone or they can be observed during functional clinical tests.

The third and last aspect related to balance is the task. Assess the goal to be achieved by the individual and how the person performs this goal are essential to screen falls. In order to approach the assessment of balance and everyday tasks, several functional clinical tests have been developed over the years. Although tests performed in a clinical setting do not fully reflect the functionality in real environments of elderly (homes, parks, sidewalks and markets), they can be useful to screen large populations, or even serve as an evaluation instrument in the rehabilitation process.

Before the choice of functional clinical test, we need to pay attention to time spent to perform the test, possible "ceiling" and "floor" effects depending on the population studied, necessary equipment and availability of physical space. It is important that the person is using its necessary compensation equipment, such as assistive devices for gait, glasses and hearing aids, in order to reproduce its functionality and ensure its best performance (Perracini & Gazzola, 2011).

The Berg Balance Scale (BBS) has 14 representative tasks of daily life, such as sitting, turning and picking up an object. Each task scores 0 to 5, according to performance, time to complete the task or need for aid. The total score varies from 0 to 56 points and the highest score refers to the best performance (Berg et al., 1992). Among community older adults, the score of 45 or less is related to prediction of falls (Thorbahn & Newton, 1996).

The Timed Up and Go (TUGT) is a widely used test to assess mobility and screen fall in elderly, because it is practical, fast and does not require a lot of equipment. In TUGT, the person is instructed to get up from an armrest chair (with high of 46 cm), walk three meters, come back and sit down again until touch the trunk support of the chair and the time taken is analyzed. It is necessary to perform the test with appropriate shoes, in usual and self-selected speed and safely. The use of assistive devices is allowed, but no physical assistance from the assessor is allowed (Perracini & Gazzola, 2011).

Bohanon (2006), in a meta-analysis study, concluded that the mean time for TUGT in elderly was 9.4 s. With advanced age, there is an increased in time spent for TUGT. For example, people aged 60-69 years spend a mean time of 9 s. On the other hand, people aged 80-99 years spent 12.7s (Bohannon, 2006). Shumway-Cook et al. (2000) recommend the time 13.5 s as cut off point to risk of falls in community-dwelling elderly.

Currently, the use of TUGT associated with a secondary task (TUGT-dual task) has been used to evaluate attentional demands on postural control in elderly. The secondary task can be motor, such as carrying a cup of water, cognitive, such as evoking name of animals or days of week and making subtraction by 3 starting from 100, or motor-cognitive. The assessor can analyze time spent, number of steps and number of right and wrong responses and compare with the performance of TUGT. According to Shumway-Cook et al. (2000), a time greater than 15 s in TUGT-dual task (secondary task: cognitive) is considered as risk of falls in community elderly.

The Dynamic Gait Index (DGI) assesses qualitatively and quantitatively the gait. It was developed with eight tasks of gait and, currently, a version of only four tasks (DGI-4) was validated by Marchetti & Whitney (2006). In this short version, the person is evaluated under gait conditions on a flat surface, with changes of speed, with horizontal movements of head and with vertical movements of head. Each item scores 0-3, with lower scores related to poorer performance. The cutoff point for risk of falls is 9 points.

The Performance Oriented Mobility Assessment (POMA) is another instrument to assess balance and gait. It can be used to screen falls in institutionalized and community elderly, with lower scores associated with poorer performances (Tinetti, 1986).

There are several tools to assess postural control in the literature. The health professional should select the most appropriate tools to its patient or its target population. It is important to note that no instrument alone is able to identify and stratify risk of falls in elderly. A comprehensive and global assessment is necessary to encompass the multiple factors involved in geriatric syndrome.

PREVENTION STRATEGIES AND LONG-TERM OUTCOMES

As falls prevention strategy, the professional should start from the prior knowledge of changes that may favor the occurrence of falls in elderly. Therefore, the concepts brought in this chapter are important to propose prevention strategies of different natures.

According to Perracini (2005), the first step of falls prevention strategy is considering the interaction between three factors: individual, environment and task. In the *individual* factor, it is important to consider deficiencies presented, who can be rehabilitated and who require compensation or replacement. In the *task* factor, it is important to identify what the demands are to carry out the specific tasks. For example, what does the individual need to remain upright and take the clothes on clothesline or wear its pants? Finally, in the *environment* factor, it is essential manipulating environmental conditions according to the interest in rehabilitation, such as simulating real situation in elevator, subway and other environments. It is necessary to identify these three factors and understand the interaction between them, and consequently professionals can propose measures that address the interventions.

In 2010, the American and British Geriatrics Society conducted a guideline for preventing falls in elderly. The guideline highlighted all seniors should be asked if they fell last year. If not, professionals should question about gait instability and presence of nearly falls. If so, it should be noted the circumstances and how often they occurred. Professionals should conduct an assessment of balance and gait. A systematic search of causal factors and risk factors (modifiable and non-modifiable) allows the proper management and prevents new events (American Geriatrics Society & British Geriatrics Society, 2010).

Given the complexity of risk factors for falls, intervention programs must address the many possible risk factors, intrinsic modifications and environmental changes (Province et al., 1995; Tinetti et al., 1996). Most of falls that lead to fractures occur indoors, especially in elderly over 80 years (Bergstrom et al., 2008). Therefore, interventions of environmental changes are necessary in elderly's home. Some studies show that environmental adaptations carried out by occupational therapists tend to be more efficient (Cumming et al., 1999; Campbell et al., 2005).

A study was conducted to evaluate if an intervention with a multidisciplinary team could reduce falls in elderly. Study participants were randomly assigned to participate in two groups. One group received a geriatric assessment followed by a home visit to diagnosis and intervention at home (control group). The other group received a geriatric assessment with recommendations and usual care to do at home. This group also received advice of possible changes in the house, facilities for any necessary modification at home and training in the use of assistive devices and mobility. After a year, the intervention group had 31% fewer falls than the control group and the intervention was more effective in a subgroup of participants who reported two or more falls during the year before recruitment for the study (Nickolaus & Bach, 2003).

Some environmental adjustments in people over 75 years with some visual impairment decreased in 24% the number of falls. The elderly were recommended to remove or alter the throw rugs on the floor mats, paint sills of the house, install grab bars, rail on the stairs and improve lighting of the house (Karlsson et al., 2013).

When the person presents intrinsic modifiable risk factors, physical interventions are recommended. A recent meta-analysis stresses that interventions for preventing falls should include a structured approach, especially in high-risk group. The authors highlighted the importance of multimodal interventions, specifically balance and strength, followed by flexibility and resistance training (Karlsson et al., 2013). Some studies show that exercise training can be performed for a long period and high frequency (Province et al., 1995).

Physical exercises, when performed in group and included two or more physical components, are effective to reduce rate of falls by 22% and risk of falls by 17%. When physical exercises are performed individually, also including two or more physical components, elderly can reduce number of falls by 34% (Karlsson et al., 2013).

In an attempt to clarify what is the best type of exercise to prevent falls in elderly, Sherrington et al. (2011) conducted a meta-analysis and established some recommendations:

- Exercises to reduce the number of falls should have moderate challenge to balance high.
- Be performed for at least two hours per week, for a continuous period - 6 months, for example.
- The exercises should be combined with exercises performed at home by the patient in order to maximize the benefits.
- The exercises can be performed in a group or individual, depending on the risk of falls of patients. If high, prefer smaller groups or individually.
- Work force and walking training should be incorporated into interventions protocols. In elderly at high risk, do not stimulate brisk walking.
- Take into consideration extrinsic factors - home adaptations, reduction of psychoactive medications (when possible).

Other forms of exercise like Tai Chi have shown effective reduction of falls. A randomized controlled study noted that only the participation of Tai Chi classes for sixteen weeks, once a week, can prevent the occurrence of falls in elderly (Voukelatos et al., 2007). The benefits can be explained as Tai Chi includes strength training and balance concomitantly (Voukelatos et al., 2007).

Another factor that may favor the occurrence of falls in elderly is the combination of different drugs. However, a prescription structured with gradual withdrawal of psychotropic medication reduced rate of falls by 66%.

In addition, changes in drug prescription may reduce rate falls by 39% (Karlsson et al., 2013).

The type of footwear can also influence risk of falling in elderly (Menant et al., 2008). A study developed a type of multifaceted intervention that included prescription orthotics for foot, advice on appropriate types of footwear even in people who could not afford to buy, a foot and ankle exercise program, a primer educational fall prevention and care in general with his foot. The intervention was effective in reducing rate of falls in community dwelling elderly with foot pain. Taking into account that intervention components are cheap and relatively simple to implement, the authors suggest the inclusion of multidisciplinary intervention to prevent falls in the elderly (Spink et al., 2011). McKiernan (2005) investigated whether a type of slip-resistant footwear was able to reduce number of falls in community elderly with a history of falls. The author noted that this type of footwear can reduce number of outdoor falls and also prevent more severe consequences related to falls.

Given these findings, it is observed that there is strong evidence that number of falls can be reduced through structured interventions. It is important that the health professional is aware of all risk factors (intrinsic and extrinsic). Therefore, this professional can make a differential diagnosis and consequently propose the best interventions measures.

Final Considerations

Falls are prevalent in older people and are a leading cause of serious injury and injury-related death, as well as a predictor of functional decline and institutionalization. Since the etiology of falls is multifactorial, the identification of the combination of risk factors in each older person needs to be done as early as possible, since it is the key to implementation of more effective prevention strategies.

The assessment of falls and the screening of people with risk for falls are complex and need to approach the interaction between environment, individual and task. Several tools area available in the literature and health professional team needs to choose the best tool for each case. We highlighted that no instrument alone is able to identify and stratify risk of falls in elderly. Therefore, a comprehensive and global assessment is necessary to encompass the complex geriatric world.

Currently there is strong evidence that both the number of falls and the number of fallers can be reduced by structured intervention. However, treating every older person is not feasible or cost effective. Therefore, the prevention is the best way to reduce the public health burden and fall-related consequences. Despite the availability of policy and practice guidelines, there are still challenges on many levels for integrating best practice falls prevention strategies into health service and therefore reducing public health impact of falls.

REFERENCES

American Geriatrics Society & British Geriatrics Society. (2010). Clinical Practice Guideline for prevention of falls. *J. Am. Geriatr. Soc.*, 1-10.

Anderson, K. (2008). Falls in the elderly. *J. R. Coll. Physicians Edinb.*, *38*, 138–143.

Australian Commission on Safety and Quality in Health Care. *Preventing falls and harm from falls in older people*: Best practice guidelines for Australian residential aged care facilities . Canberra, 2009.

Berg, K. O., Wood-Dauphinee, S. L., Williams, J. I. & Maki, B. (1992). Measuring balance in the elderly: validation of an instrument. *Can. J. Public Health*, *83*(2), 7-11.

Bergström, U., Björnstig, U. Stenlund, H., et al. (2008). Fracture mechanisms and fracture pattern in men and women aged 50 years and older: a study of a 12-year population-based injury register, Umeå, Sweden. *Osteoporos. Int.*, *19*, 1267–73.

Bohannon, R. W. (2006). Reference values for the Timed Up and Go test: a descriptive meta-analysis. *J. Geriatr. Phys. Ther.*, *29*(2), 64-68.

Buracchio, T. et al. (2010). The trajectory of gait speed preceding mild cognitive impairment. *Arch. Neurol.*, *67*, 980-986.

Campbell, A. J. et al. (2005). Randomised controlled trial of prevention of falls in people aged > or =75 with severe visual impairment: the VIP trial. *BMJ*, *331*, 817.

Chang, J. et al. (2004). Interventions for the prevention of falls in older adults: systematic review and meta-analysis of randomised clinical trials. *BMJ*, *328*(7441), 680.

Chiu, A. Y., Au-Yeung, S. S. & Lo, S. K. (2003). A comparison of four functional tests in discriminating fallers from non-fallers in older people. *Disabil. Rehabil.*, *25*(1), 45-50.

Cumming, R. G. et al. (1999). Home visits by an occupational therapist for assessment and modification of environmental hazards: a randomized trial of falls prevention. *J. Am. Geriatr. Soc.*, *47*, 1397–402.

Delbaere, K., Close, J. C. T., Mikolaizak, A. S., Sachdev, P. S., Brodaty, H. & Lord, S. R. (2010). The Falls Efficacy Scale International (FES-I). A comprehensive longitudinal validation study. *Age Ageing*, *39*(2), 210–216.

Evans, D., Hodgkinson, B., Lambert, L. & Wood, J. (2001). Falls risk factors in the hospital setting: a systematic review. *Int. J. Nurs. Pract.*, *7*(1), 38-45.

Fleming, J., Matthews, F. E. & Brayne, C. (2008). CC75C Study Collaboration. Falls in advanced old age: recalled falls and prospective follow-up of over-90-year-olds in the Cambridge City over-75s Cohort study. *BMC Geriatr.*, *8*, 6.

Franssen, E. H., Souren, L. E. M., Torossian, C. L. & Reisberg, B. (1999). Equilibrium and Limb coordination in mild cognitive impairment and mild Alzheimer´s disease. *J. Am. Geriatr. Soc.*, *47*, 463- 469.

Hall, C. B. et al. (2000). A change point model for estimating the onset of cognitive decline in preclinical Alzheimer's disease. *Stat. Med.*, *19*, 1555–66.

Healey, F., Scobie, S., Oliver, D., Pryce, A., Thomson, R. & Glampson, B. (2008). Falls in English and Welsh hospitals: A national observational study based on retrospective analysis of 12 months of patient safety incident reports. *Qual. Saf. Health Care*, *17*(6), 424-430.

Imamura, T. (2000). Fall-related injuries in dementia with Lewy bodies (DLB) and Alzheimer´s disease. *Eur. J. Neurol.*, *7*, 77-79.

Karlsson, M. K., Vonschewelov, T., Karlsson, C., Coster, M. & Rosengen, B. E. Prevention of falls in the elderly: a review. *Scand. J. Public Health.*, *41*, 442-454.

Kato, E. M. & Radanovic, M. (2007). Alterações motoras nas demências. In: Kato, E. M. ; Radanovic, M. *Fisioterapia nas demências*. 1 ed. São Paulo: Atheneu, 25-37,

Kelsey, J. L., Procter-Gray, E., Nguyen, U. S. D., Li, W., Kiel, D. P. & Hannan, M. T. (2010). Footwear and falls in the home among older individuals in the Mobilize Boston Study. *Footwear Sci.*, *2*(3): 123–129.

Koepsell, T. et al. (2004). Footwear style and risk of falls in older adults. *J. Am. Geriatr. Soc.*, *52*(9), 1495-501.

Kwan, M. M., Close, J. C., Wong, A. K. & Lord, E. R. (2011). Falls Incidence, Risk Factors, and Consequences in Chinese Older People: A Systematic Review. *J. Am. Geriatr. Soc.*, *59*(3), 536-543.

Liu-Ambrose, P. T. et al. (2008). Mild cognitive impairment increases falls risk in older community-dwelling women. *Phys. Ther.*, *88*(12), 1482-1491.

Luukinen, H., Herala, M., Koski, K., Honkanen, R., Laippala, P. & Kivelä S. L. (2000). Fracture risk associated with a fall according to type of fall among the elderly. *Osteoporos. Int.*, *11*(7), 631-634.

Luukinen, H., Koski, K., Laippala, P. & Kivela, S. L. (1997). Factors predicting fractures during falling impacts among home-dwelling older adults. *J. Am. Geriatr. Soc.*, *45*(11), 1302-1309.

Marchetti, G. F. & Whitney, S. L. (2006). Construction and validation of the 4-item Dynamic Gait Index. *Phys. Ther.*, *86*(12), 1651-60.

McKiernan, F. E. (2005). A simple gait-stabilizing device reduces outdoor falls and non serious injurious falls in fall prone older people during the winter. *J. Am. Geriatr. Soc.*, *53*, 943–7.

Menant, J. et al. (2008). Optimizing footwear for older people at risk of falls. *J. Rehabil. Res. Dev.*, *45*(8), 1167-81.

Montero-Odasso, M., Muir, S. W. & Speechley, M. (2012). Dual-task complexity affects gait in people with mild cognitive impairment: the interplay between gait variability, dual tasking, and risk of falls. *Arch. Phys. Med. Rehabil.*, *93*, 293-299.

National Ageing Research Institute. *An Analysis of Research on Preventing Falls and Falls Injury in Older People:* Community, residential care and hospital settings. Canberra, 2004.

Nevitt, M. C., Cummings, S. R., Kidd, S. & Black, D. (1989). Risk factors for recurrent nonsyncopal falls: a prospective study. *JAMA*, *261*(18), 2663-2668.

Oliver, D. & Healy, F. (2009). Falls risk prediction tools for hospital inpatients: Do they work? *Nurs. Times*, *105*(7), 18-21.

Peel, N. M. (2011). Epidemiology of Falls in Older Age. *Can. J. Aging*, *30*(1), 7-19.

Peeters, G. & Lips, P. (2009). Fall risk: the clinical relevance of falls and how to integrate fall risk with fracture risk. *Best Pract. Res. Clin. Rheumatol.*, *23*(6), 797–804.

Perracini, M. R. Prevenção e manejo de quedas. In: Ramos, L. R. *Guia de Geriatria e Gerontologia*. Barueri, SP: Manole, 2005.

Perracini, M. R., Gazzola, J. M. Balance em idosos. In: Perracini, M. R., Fló, C. M. *Funcionalidade e envelhecimento*. Rio de Janeiro, RJ: Guanabara Koogan, 2011.

Perracini, M. R. & Ramos, L. R. (2002). Fatores associados a quedas em uma coorte de idosos residentes na comunidade. *Rev. Saúde Públ.*, *36*(6), 709-16.

Province, M. A. et al. (1995). The effects of exercise on falls in elderly patients. A preplanned meta-analysis of the FICSIT Trials. Frailty and injuries: cooperative studies of intervention techniques. *JAMA*, *273*, 1341–7.

Rodriguez, J. G. et al. (1995). A standardized instrument to assess hazards for falls in the home of older persons. *Accid Anal Prev*, *27*(5), 625-31. Rubenstein, L. (2006). Falls in older people: epidemiology, risk factors and strategies for prevention. *Age Aging*, *35*(2), 37-41.

Sheridan, P. L. & Hausdorff J. M. (2007). The role of higher - level cognitive function in gait: Executive dysfunction contributes to fall risk in Alzheimer's disease. *Dement. Geriatr. Cogn. Disord.*, *24*, 125-137.

Shumway-Cook, A., Brauer, S. & Woollacott, M. (2000). Predicting the probability for falls in community-dwelling older adults using the Timed Up & Go test. *Phys. Ther.*, *80*(9), 896-903.

Shumway-Cook, A. & Horak, F. B. (1986). Assessing the influence of sensory interaction on balance. *Phys. Ther.*, *66*(10), 1548-1550.

Siu, K. C., Chou, L. S., Mayr, U., Donkelaar, P. V. & Woollacott, M. H. (2008). Does inability to allocate attention contribute to balance constraints during gait in older adults? *J. Gerontol.*, *63*(12), 1364-1369.

Spink, M. J., Menz, H. B. & Fotoohabadi, M. R., et al. (2011). Effectiveness of a multifaceted podiatry intervention to prevent falls in community dwelling older people with disabling foot pain: randomized controlled trial. *BMJ*, 342:d3411.

Stel, V. S., Pluijm, S. M., Deeg, D. J., Smit, J. H., Bouter, L. M. & Lips, P. (2003). A classification tree for predicting recurrent falling in community-dwelling older persons. *J. Am. Geriatr. Soc.*, *51*(10), 1356–1364.

Stubbs, B., Binnekade, T., Eggermont, L., Sephery, A. A. & Patchay, S., Schofield, P. (2014). Pain and the risk for falls in community-dwelling older adults: systematic review and meta-analysis. *Arch. Phys. Med. Rehabil.*, *95*(1), 175-187.

Tencer, A. F. et al. (2004). Biomechanical properties of shoes and risk of falls in older adults. *J. Am. Geriatr. Soc.*, *52*(11), 1840-46.

Thorbahn, L. D. B. & Newton, R. A. (1996). Use of the Berg Balance test to predict falls in elderly persons. *Phys. Ther.*, *76*(6), 576:83.

Tinetti, M. E. (1986). Performance-oriented assessment of mobility problems in elderly patients. *J. Am. Geriatr. Soc.*, *34*(2), 119-126.

Tinetti, M. E., McAvay, G. & Claus, E. (1996). Does multiple risk factor reduction explain the reduction in fall rate in the Yale FICSIT Trial? Frailty and injuries cooperative studies of intervention techniques. *Am. J. Epidemiol.*, *144*, 389–99.

Tinetti, M. E., Speechley, M. & Ginter, S. F. (1998). Risk factors for falls among community-dwelling elderly. *N. Engl. J. Med.*, *319*(26), 1701-7.

Umphred, D. A. (2004). *Reabilitação Neurológica*. 4 ed. Barueri, SP: Manole.

Van Iersel, M. B., Kessels, R. P. C., Bloem, B. R., Verbeek, A. L. M. & Olde Rikkert, M. G. M. (2008). Executive functions are associated with gait and balance in community-living elderly people. *J. Gerontol. A Biol. Sci. Med. Sci.*, *63*(12), 1344-1349.

Verghese, J. et al. (2007). Quantitative gait dysfunction and risk of cognitive decline and dementia. *J. Neurol. Neurosurg. Psychiatry*, *78*, 929-935.

Voukelatos, A. et al. (2007). A randomized, controlled trial of tai chi for the prevention of falls: the Central Sydney tai chi trial. *J. Am. Geriatr. Soc.*, *55*, 1185–1191.

Whitney, S. L., Wrisley, D. M., Marchetti, G. F., Gee, M. A., Redfern, M. S. & Furman, J. M. (2005). Clinical measurement of Sit-to-Stand performance in people with balance disorders: validity of data for the Five-Times-Sit-to-Stand Test. *Phys. Ther.*, *85*(10), 1034-1045.

World Health Organization. *Older persons in emergency*: an active aging perspective. Geneva, 2008.

World Health Organization. *WHO Global Report on Falls Prevention in Older Age*. Geneva, 2007.

Yardley, L., Beyer, N., Hauer, K., Kempen, G., Piot-Ziegler, C. & Todd, C. (2005). Development and initial validation of the Falls Efficacy Scale – International (FES-I). *Age Ageing*, *34*(6), 614-19.

In: Accidental Falls
Editor: Brenda Evans

ISBN: 978-1-63483-228-1

Chapter 2

DETERMINANTS OF ACCIDENTAL FALLS AND FALL-RELATED INJURIES: RECOMMENDATIONS FOR FALLS AND FALL-RELATED INJURIES PREVENTION SET ON THE ANALYSIS OF A THEORETICAL DYNAMIC SYSTEM INVOLVING THE OLDER ADULT, THE ENVIRONMENT, AND THE TASK PERFORMANCE

Catarina Lino Neto Pereira and Ana Isabel Carvalho Cruz-Ferreira

Departamento de Desporto e Saúde; Escola de Ciências e Tecnologia; Universidade de Évora; Research Center in Sports Sciences, Health and Human Development (CIDESD); Évora, Portugal

ABSTRACT

This work aims to provide easy and practical recommendations for falls and fall-related injuries prevention set on the analysis of a theoretical dynamic system involving the subject (older adult), the environment, and the task performance.

In accordance with this system, accidental falls occur while performing physical activities/tasks. In the absence of movement the probability of falling will be almost zero. However, immobility decreases the subject´s ability of performance. The fall usually occurs when the demands of a given task exceed the subject's ability. The demands of a task are determined by its difficulty and by environmental conditions. In a hostile environment, the demands of a given task increase. As result, the task demands may exceed the subject's ability causing a fall.

The ability to perform daily tasks without falling tends to decline with age due to associated frailty (notably the increased morbidities and the diminished physical, sensorial, and neural fitness). However, falls may also be a problem before the age of 60 years. The main immediate consequence of a fall is injury, which may be fatal. Another possible short-term consequence is an increased fear of falling that often conducts to a loss of independence while performing daily tasks and, consequently, leads to a decline in the subject's ability.

It was observed that the determinant factor for the rupture of this system balance (resulting in falls and fall-related injuries) in older adults is the subject, namely his/her condition of frailty. As the subject becomes more fragile and as the risk of intrinsic factors increases, their susceptibility to extrinsic factors rises, especially with regard to environmental hazards. Thereafter, the subject's likelihood of falling and injuring increases. However, a good level of physical fitness can also increase the threat of falling and injuring, because fitter people are more confidence in performing more demanding tasks and in more hazardous environments. Thereby, they expose themselves to more dangerous situations.

Given the above and reporting recent research findings, the primary recommendations for fall and fall-related injuries prevention are the following:

- A healthy lifestyle, in order to avoid co-morbidities or, at least, to minimize its effects.
- The reduction of environmental hazards, principally when fitness decreases and frailty increases, and the restraint of difficult tasks in hazardous environments.
- The practice at least 1,150 MET-min.wk^{-1} of physical activity, with no more than 500 MET-min.wk^{-1} (~60 min. wk^{-1}) of vigorous physical activity (due to associated hazards). For example a combination of 1 hour of walking, 2 hours of moderate physical activity (such as carrying light loads or bicycling at a regular pace) and 20 minutes of vigorous physical activity (such as heavy lifting, digging, aerobics, or fast bicycling) per week, what computes ~1,150 MET-min.wk^{-1}.

- The implementation of exercise programs to prevent physical fitness loss, especially balance. Further, muscle strength and gait exercises may be particularly relevant for less fit and frail people.
- The performance of functional exercises that mimic everyday life tasks and promote self-confidence.
- Regarding women, special attention must be taken because they tend to be more fragile. Regarding men, special attention must be taken because they tend to expose themselves to more hazardous situations.

1. INTRODUCTION

Maintaining quality of life throughout the aging process expressed as independent functioning and healthy status is a major concern of each subject. This has also become a key issue of modern societies, given the current demographic explosion of the third age (Eurostat, 2014). In 2012, the average life expectancy at birth of the global population was 70 years and the healthy life expectancy at birth was 62 globally (WHO, 2014). In the United States, life expectancy at birth rose 0.4 years from 2003 to 2004, reaching a record of 77.8 years (Minino, Heron, Murphy, & Kochanek, 2007); in Germany, life expectancy increased from 75 years, in 1990, to 80 years, in 2008 (WHO, 2010); in Portugal, it is expected that the number of people over 65 years will increase from 17% to 32% between 2008 and 2060 and that the percentage of those over 80 years will rise from 4% to 13% during the same period (INE;IP, 2009).

Successful aging implies not only more years of life (quantity) but also quality of life: the absence of chronic health conditions and the ability to function effectively, both physically and mentally (Britton, Shipley, Singh-Manoux, & Marmot, 2008). Successful older adults continue on living independently in their own homes (Nosraty, Jylha, Raittila, & Lumme-Sandt, 2015).

The occurrence of falls increases with age, and it is estimated that at least 30% of people aged 65 or older who live in a community fall at least once a year (Tinetti, Speechley, & Ginter, 1988). However, falls may be a problem before the age of 60 (Nitz & Choy, 2008). The risk of both falls and fall-related injuries, and loss of independence coexist (Barrett-Connor, Weiss, McHorney, Miller, & Siris, 2009; Pereira, 2011; Tak, Kuiper, Chorus, & Hopman-Rock, 2014; Tinetti et al., 1988); with falls in the elderly being pointed as a major reason for lower quality of life, loss of independence, institutionalization or death (Alamgir, Muazzam, & Nasrullah, 2012; Donald & Bulpitt, 1999; Robbins, Biggs, & Cauley, 2006). Around 30% to 50% of falls leads to minor injuries and 5% to 10% result to major injuries, namely hip fractures (Goldacre, Roberts, & Yeates, 2002). Beyond the injuries, falls lead to fear of falling, loss of independence, and death in a third of those older adults (Ambrose, Paul, & Hausdorff, 2013). In fact, falls are the major cause of death related to mechanical injuries in the elderly (Alamgir et al., 2012). The direct costs alone from fall-related injuries are at a staggering 0.1% and up to 1.5% of all healthcare expenses in United States and Europe, respectively. Given the aging of population and the consequent increase at-risk sample, it is expected that these costs will increase (Ambrose et al., 2013).

Not only the most obvious consequences of fall-related injuries, but also the fear of falling lead to the restriction of normal activities among a large percentage of the older adults (Denkinger, Lukas, Nikolaus, & Hauer, 2015; Fuzhong, Fisher, Harmer, MacAuley, & Wilson, 2003; Zijlstra, Haastregt, Eijk, & Kempen, 2005). Furthermore, depression, feeling of helplessness, and social isolation also contribute to disability in the performance of activities of daily living (Lenze et al., 2007). The activities of daily living include: (i) basic activities of hygiene, personal care, and getting around inside; (ii) instrumental activities, that is, activities necessary for living in the community such as using transportation, shopping, preparing meals, and paying bills; and (iii) advanced activities comprising more demanding and non-survival type of activities that enrich life, namely social, religious or leisure activities (Reuben & Solomon, 1989; Spector & Fleishman, 1998). Most of the risk factors for loss of independence in the performance of activities of daily living and for falls and fall-related injuries are common, such as age (Hardy & Gill, 2005), reduced physical function/fitness (Pereira, Baptista, & Infante, 2014; Rikli & Jones, 2001), gait disorders (Brach & VanSwearingen, 2002), poor body composition (Vasquez, Batsis, Germain, & Shaw, 2014), and health conditions (Jung, Ostbye, & Park, 2006; Stessman, Hammerman-Rozenberg, Maaravi, Azoulai, & Cohen, 2005).

Physical activity is one of the main factors known to help maintain independence (Hardy & Gill, 2005; Paterson & Warburton, 2010; Pynnonen, Tormakangas, Heikkinen, Rantanen, & Lyyra, 2012; Stessman et al., 2005; Tak et al., 2014) and to be effective in fall prevention (Sherrington et al., 2008) and fall-related injuries (Kannus, 2006; Karinkanta et al., 2009; Pereira & Baptista, 2012). Many different types of exercise programs have been implemented in older adults and have proved being addressed to the challenges of aging successfully, which covers fall-related injury prevention (Achour et al., 2011; Cruz-Ferreira, Marmeleira, Formigo, Gomes, & Fernandes, 2015; Kannus, Sievanen, Palvanen, Jarvinen, & Parkkari, 2005; Marmeleira et al., 2009; Rose, 2008).

Although measures to prevent the occurrence of falls and their consequences are known, the knowledge that enables the implementation of effective strategies to large populations is still insufficient. This work aims to provide easy and practical recommendations for falls and fall-related injuries prevention set on the analysis of a theoretical dynamic system involving the subject (older adult), the environment, and the task performance.

2. Fall and Fall-related Injuries: A Theoretical Approach

In order to outline effective recommendations for fall and fall-related injuries preventions, we propose a theoretical approach examining the problem of falls and fall-related injuries. The model was developed by Pereira (Pereira, 2011) based on several researches (Association of Emergency Medical Technicians, 2003; Davids, Glazier, Araujo, & Bartlett, 2003; Glazier & Davids, 2009). The following text shows the model organized by three items: the fall, the injury, and the maintenance of independence in older adults.

2.1. The Fall

A fall is an accident in which a person "suddenly and involuntary comes to rest upon the ground or on a surface lower than the original station" (Hogan et al., 2001; Oliver, Britton, Seed, Martin, & Hopper, 1997). The phenomenon involves the existence of three interacting components or constrains: the subject, the task, and the environment (Figure 1). This theoretical model is described below and is centered on these three components.

With their capacity for accomplishment or performance of tasks, able people usually live in a more or less harmonious environment that allows them to carry out everyday tasks without great difficulty and in safety. The occurrence of falls will depend on the capability of the subject to maintain a balance between their ability of performance and the demands of the tasks. An accident (fall) will occur when the demands of one particular task exceed the ability of the person to perform that task. These demands depend on the difficulty of the task itself and also on the environment: in a hostile environment, the demands of a given task increase (Pereira, 2011)

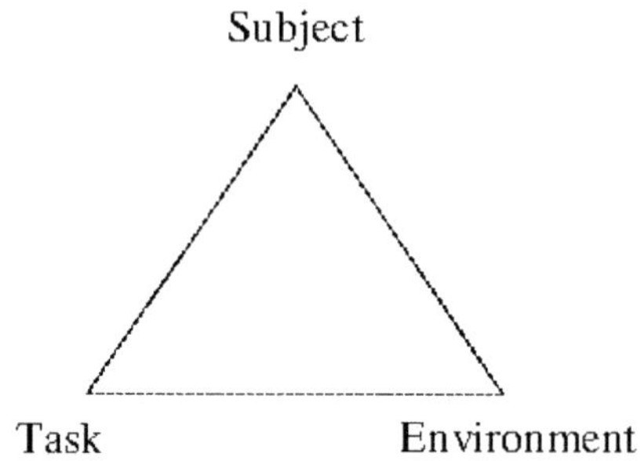

Figure 1. The three components involved in the fall.

A fall may occur when there is an imbalance between the ability of the subject (depending on their function/capacity) and the demands of the task and/or the environment, specifically when one or several of the following events occur:

- the demand of the task exceeds the subject's ability for performance;
- the environment evolves in such an unfavorable way that the normal ability of the subject for performance is insufficient to confront environmental difficulties and simultaneously to carry out the task;
- the subject's ability for performance decreases and the demands of the task and/or the environmental difficulties are not successfully overcome, even in the case of normal daily tasks.

The fall may not occur when:

- the subject's function and consequently ability is high enough to enable them to carry out any task in a normal environment or those with a degree of difficulty or some demands;
- there is a reduction in one or more of the functional abilities of the subject; however, this reduction is compensated by other abilities that still allow them to successfully perform the task;
- the demands of the task do not challenge the ability of the subject to perform, in an environment of normal difficulty;

- the environment is so favorable that it enables the task to be successfully carried out;
- there is no task to be carried out, hence there is no difficulty.

Therefore, the variability of functional performance must be considered since, in the performance of functional movement, different degrees of freedom enable different solutions for the successful accomplishment of a given task (Davids et al., 2003). The variability of movement helps the subject to adapt to the unique constraints (associated with the subject, the task, and the environment) successfully (without falling).

When people age, their ability to perform tasks is expected to decrease because, besides demonstrating a higher level of morbidity, functional ability naturally decreases with age (de Rekeneire et al., 2003; Gill, Gahbauer, Lin, Han, & Allore, 2013; Rikli & Jones, 1999). As functionality decreases, people are increasingly less able to deal with less demanding situations (Gitlin et al., 2006), either in terms of the environment or the task. Furthermore, as aging advances, human movement systems tend to be characterized by a loss in complexity and also the decrease of movement variability resulting in poor adaptation to environmental changes (Davids et al., 2003; Hundrup, Ekholm, Hoidrup, Davidsen, & Obel, 2005). In fact, the aging process contributes to a progressively precarious balance between the three components of the system and, as the chance of the rupture of this balance increases, the probability of the occurrence of falls rises (Pereira, 2011). Moreover, older adult are not usually aware of their predisposition to falls and injuries, and consequently are not able to identify inherent risk factors with regard to falls; the risk becomes obvious only after the occurrence of injury or disability (Braun, 1998).

When the ability of performance is drastically reduced, older adults may lose even the ability for meeting the demands of everyday tasks (Gitlin et al., 2006; Li et al., 2006). In this case, a fall may occur during the performance of such tasks, which nevertheless present a very low degree of difficulty, and not only during the performance of more demanding tasks (Gill, Zou, Jones, & Speechley, 2008; Gitlin et al., 2006; Stewart et al., 2005).

The loss of functionality in the older adult is accompanied by a decrease in their capacity for carrying out tasks in less favorable environments (for example, neglecting toys on the floor that create an obstacle to reaching the telephone); this is why an understanding of the role of extrinsic risk factors for falling and/or environment hazards with different degrees of functionality is so important (Bath & Morgan, 1999; Tinetti, 2003; Tinetti & Speechley, 1989).

Therefore, the ability for accomplishing tasks and, accordingly, the ability for carrying out tasks without falling depends on several ability factors: somatic, physical, sensorial, information analysis, and response among others (Aoyama, Suzuki, Onishi, & Kuzuya, 2011; Bateni, Zecevic, MacIlroy, & Maki, 2004; Rogers, Rogers, Takeshima, & Islam, 2003; Stewart et al., 2005; van Heuvelen et al., 2005). If the task and/or the environment are not excessively demanding, a high level of ability regarding some factors will probably compensate for a lower level of ability for others, allowing the subject to successfully perform a given task. However, the gradual nature of the aging process (Vitetta & Anton, 2007) means that rupture in the balance between the three components of the system ends only with death.

The components of falling will be detail analyzed in order to find which and how the components involved in this model can be manipulated to counteract or delay the tendency for rupture and how this can be achieved.

2.2. The Components of the Fall

2.2.1. The Task

The first attempt to avoid falls and fall-related injuries is inactivity: if the subject does not move and lies or sits without doing anything, consequently not performing any physical activity or task, the probability of falling will be practically zero. However, if he does not perform any physical activity, his functional level will decline and his ability to perform will decrease drastically (Nelson et al., 2007). Consequently, any task (e.g. to go to the bathroom) may be so demanding to the older adult that he may be not able to successfully meet and a fall may occur during the performance of the task.

The risk of accidental fall and injuries will depend on the exposure to the hazard that is involved on the activity participation (Wijlhuizen, Chorus, & Hopman-Rock, 2010). On one side, physical activity improves physical fitness; on the other side, physical activity exposes the subject to the hazards. Hence, either low or high levels of physical activity have been associated with an increased risk of falling and injury, with regard to the exposure to hazards involved and with regard to the subject level of fit (Chan et al., 2007; Etman, Wijlhuizen, van Heuvelen, Chorus, & Hopman-Rock, 2012; Gill et al., 2008; Gregg, Cauley, Seeley, Ensrud, & Bauer, 1998; Peeters et al., 2010; Wijlhuizen et al., 2010). Current research studies recommend that interventions designed to prevent falls and injuries should promote physical activity/exercise (Carter et al., 2002; Liu-Ambrose et al., 2005; Nelson et al.,

2007). Pereira and her collaborators (Pereira et al., 2014) observed that increasing 500 MET-min/wk in physical activity (i.e., ~90 min of moderated physical activity such as carrying light loads or bicycling at a regular pace; in addition to 40 min of walking) leads directly to a decrease in the likelihood of falling (by 86%). This increase in physical activity would lead to a further indirectly decrease in the risk of falling by increasing physical fitness (Chodzko-Zajko et al., 2009). Pereira and her collaborators (Pereira et al., 2014) also observed that vigorous physical activity (such as heavy lifting, digging, aerobics or fast bicycling) reduced the risk of falls by increasing activity, but only up to the threshold of 500 MET-min/wk. Above this threshold, vigorous physical activity only would increase the risk of falls (5% for each additional 100 MET-min/wk) (Pereira et al., 2014); this is most likely because, at a higher physical activity levels (e.g. farming or tennis), tasks are more demanding (Glazier & Davids, 2009) and the propensity for falls is greater. Therefore, a physical activity of at least 1,125 MET-min/wk with no more than 500 MET-min/wk (i.e., less than ~1 hr/wk) of vigorous physical activity significantly reduced falls. For example, a combination of 1 hour of walking, 2 hours of moderate physical activity, and 20 minutes of vigorous physical activity per week, which computes ~1,150 MET-min.wk-1.

2.2.2. The Environment

Environmental control is always an important factor because, with aging, the older adults tend to neglect their houses, gardens, and their general environment, living sometimes in the midst of very hazardous conditions (Lamontagne, Levesque, Gingras, Maurice, & Verreault, 2004). An external agent, who provides care for them, may be required to draw up an inventory of risk situations and find the best solution for each subject (Gitlin et al., 2006; Lamontagne et al., 2004). This may involve simply installing supporting bars in the bathtub, replacing the chair stood on to change light bulbs with a small ladder, or relocating cooking utensils in a more accessible place.

As the number of hazardous conditions increases, the threat of falling usually increases (Pluijm et al., 2006; Tinetti et al., 1988). Nevertheless, the probability of falling is reduced when older people are healthier and fitter; so that healthier and fitter older adults do not fall as often as younger less healthier and unfit people, even when living in environments that are more hazardous (Pereira et al., 2014). These results suggest that extrinsic risk factors (environment) contribute to falls, particularly in the presence of intrinsic risk factors (co-morbidities, decreased balance, and poor body composition), despite age (Pereira et al., 2014).

Tinetti and her collaborator (Tinetti & Speechley, 1989) identified 34 environmental hazard, including (i) indoor hazards (e.g. bad lighting, slippery floors, loose rugs, telephone cables, and other objects; ladders, stairways with steep steps, without walls and/or handrails, kitchens with difficult access to utensils and movable tables, bathrooms without tub handrails, shower and toilet and non-skid mat in tub or shower, bed too high or too low); (ii) outdoor hazards (e.g. bad lighting, uneven pavements, streets, paths, repair works, obstacles, slippery floors), (iii) the presence of animals, and (iv) footwear (e.g. high heels, poor adherence to the foot, slippery).

This list allows the identification of environmental hazards and may be used by older adults and caregivers for changing the environment and making it safe. These changes must take in account the older adults' frailty with regard to the exposure to hazards involved (Etman et al., 2012; Wijlhuizen et al., 2010). Older adults and caregivers should be aware that the likelihood of falling decreases 12.2% for each environment hazard that is removed (Pereira et al., 2014).

2.2.3. The Subject

Although the aging process cannot be stopped, some measures can be implemented to reduce its negative effects (Crimmins, Hayward, Hagedorn, Saito, & Brouard, 2009; Hashimoto et al., 2010; Yokoya, Demura, & Sato, 2009). Getting glasses or a hearing aid can counteract the natural loss of capacity of the visual and auditory systems (Vouriot et al., 2004). At a proprioceptive level, it may be more difficult to mitigate the loss of sensory capacity, but the use of suitable foot-ware with non-slip soles, for example, may be significant in preventing falls (Menant, Steele, Menz, Munro, & Lord, 2008). Additionally, medication and treatments may be prescribed for incapacity caused either by the natural degradation of the organism or illnesses (Cooper & Burfield, 2009). However, it is important to prevent the side-effects of both medication and treatments, such as the effects of anti-depressants that decrease attention and may contribute to a fall (Coutinho, Fletcher, Bloch, & Rodrigues, 2008).

Another level of intervention involves physical exercise for the maintenance of functional abilities. Physical activity/exercise improves physical fitness and body composition (Chodzko-Zajko et al., 2009), preventing the reduction of functional abilities and skills (Achour et al., 2011; Yokoya et al., 2009). Further, physical activity prevents or decreases the effects of illness (Rose, 2008), and health conditions are the most important determinant of falls and physical functioning (Pereira, 2011). Although it was not expected, some studies (Pereira, Baptista, & Infante, 2013; Pereira et al., 2014) showed that age was not a significant risk factor for falls under favorable conditions of health, body composition, and physical fitness. Thereby, a high physical fitness prevents the occurrence of falls, namely a good level of motor coordination, balance, agility, muscle strength, flexibility, and aerobic endurance. Poor balance and body composition (especially lean body mass) were pointed as the main physical fitness determinants of the risk of falling in community dwelling older adults (Pereira et al., 2013; Pereira et al., 2014).

The maintenance of gait pattern and attention capacity is also crucial for successfully meeting the demands inherent to the performance of specific motor tasks (the dual-task paradigm) (Cornillon et al., 2002; Ojha, Kern, Lin, & Winstein, 2009; Pluijm et al., 2006; Rogers, Rogers, Chaparro, Stumpfhauser, & Halcomb, 2003). Therefore, the engagement in physical activity programs has shown to be one of the most effective strategies to prevent falls (Nyman & Victor, 2012).

Several studies reported a different susceptibility to falls depending on gender, showing that women are more susceptible to falls than men (Chu, Chi, & Chiu, 2005; de Rekeneire et al., 2003). Pereira and collaborators (Pereira & Baptista, 2012; Pereira et al., 2013) concluded that this susceptibility could be explained by women's poorer health and physical fitness comparing to men's. These researchers also founded that when similar conditions of health and physical fitness were considered for both men and women, men were twice more likely to fall than women. These findings were consistent with the statement that men reported a higher percentage of falls than women when performing risky and high-difficulty tasks, but a lower percentage of falls when performing harmless habitual tasks (Pereira et al., 2013; Pereira et al., 2014).

In conclusion, effective interventions must target a healthy physical fitness, focusing particularly on body composition and balance and drawing special attention to women, because their conditions tend to be more fragile, and to men, because they tend to expose themselves to situations of greater risk (Pereira, 2011).

2.3. The Injury

The most obvious consequence of falls is injury (Bialoszewski et al., 2008; Yeo, Lee, Lim, Quek, & Ooi, 2009). In this work, an injury is considered to be an infirmity that involves the necessary interaction of three components (Association of Emergency Medical Technicians, 2003). Figure 2 illustrates this disease triangle comprising:

- an agent that causes the infirmity (uncontrolled energy released by an object depending on the velocity, shape, material, and time of exposition);
- a host in which the agent may reside;
- an environment in which the agent and the host come together.

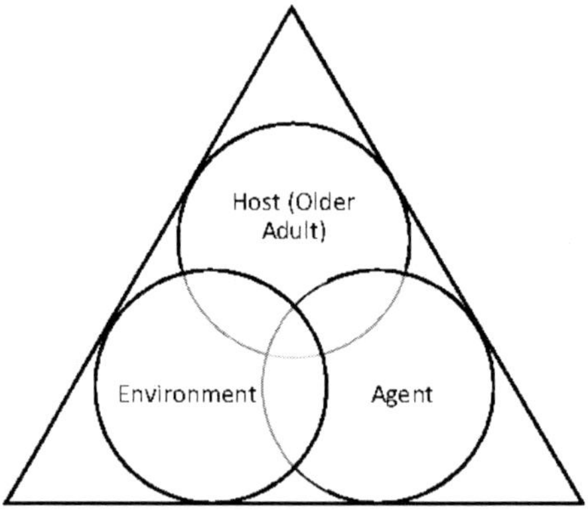

Figure 2. Disease triangle (adapted from Association of Emergency Medical Technicians ACoS. 2003).

The fall is a serious problem because it is the determining factor for the fall-related injury (Douglas, Mehan, Collins, Smith, & McKenzie, 2009; Pereira et al., 2014; Yeo et al., 2009). Injury severity depends on:

- the environment that enables the interaction between the agent and the host;
- the injury agent, for example the surface type where the mechanical aggression occurs;

- host susceptibility (which is increased in the older adult), for example body tissue resistance and the ability of the subject to decrease the impact of the fall (Association of Emergency Medical Technicians, 2003; Laing & Robinovitch, 2009; Pluijm, 2001).

Injuries severity range from simple abrasions or contusions to bone fractures, and depend on the location in the body (Ojo, O'Connor, Kim, Ciardiello, & Bonadies, 2009; Stevens, Thomas, Teh, & Greenspan, 2009; Yeo et al., 2009). The major health cost is allocated to fractures (McLean, Day, & Dalton) that may occur in any bone of the skeleton. The most frequent are humeral, fist, pelvis and, especially, hip fractures that are positively correlated with age and usually result from the combined effects of osteoporosis and the fall itself (Kannus et al., 2005; Pereira, Vogelaere, & Baptista, 2008). Despite its severity, adapting the environment, destroying the agent, or strengthening the host can control the injury.

2.3.1. Injury Prevention

Preventive interventions should promote every action that decreases the occurrence and probability of falls (Gillespie et al., 2009). As it is impossible to completely exclude the possibility of falls because they may occur in any place and any object may unexpectedly act as an injury agent (e.g. a chair, the bathtub, stairs, or the floor where the mechanical aggression occurs), the priority is to decrease the risk of a fall. This issue may be achieved by controlling the environment, the agent, and the host, as explained above.

The identification of environmental hazards and the implementation of measures to control hazards (the use of a bath chair in the bathtub, for example) or to eliminate them (removing dangerous objects from the environment) may prevent injury or at least decrease the severity of injuries (Gitlin et al., 2006; Lamontagne et al., 2004). As reported bellow, the list proposed by Tinetti and collaborator (Tinetti & Speechley, 1989) identifying environmental hazards may be used to this end.

The reduction of host susceptibility to the agent is also a primordial option. However, this is an attempt to counteract the natural trend towards aging (Vitetta & Anton, 2007). Older adults gradually lose their reflexes and functional abilities, which may lead to an increase in the amount of uncontrolled energy released by the aggressive agent. They also have less tissue elasticity and are consequently more susceptible to tissue rupture (Cadarette et al., 2000; Wang, Li, Shen, & Agrawal, 2003). Moreover, age is associated with the osteoporosis phenomenon, the main reason for decline in bone resistance and the consequently increase in fracture susceptibility (Brown & Josse, 2002; Kanis, 2002), which is higher in women (Kannus et al., 2005).

Therefore, there must be a balance between (i) the performance of activities, that decrease the host susceptibility, and (ii) the risk associated with the performance of any activity, that potentially allow the interaction between the host and the agent (especially if the involved tasks are high demanding and are performed in a hazard environment).

Gill and collaborators (Gill et al., 2008) concluded that injurious falls were associated with higher recreational physical activity and with lower subsequent household physical activity. On another hand, Li and collaborators (Li et al., 2006) observed that people who reported more leisure-time physical activity had a higher risk for outdoor falls, and people who were in poorer health had a greater risk for indoor falls. These results may be explained by the higher self-exposure to the agent made by fitter people, and by the higher susceptibility of the frail people to the injury agent (Kelsey et al., 2010; Pereira, 2011).

Despite the fact that physical activity enables falls occurrence, as already mentioned, being active decreases the risk of severe fall-related injuries (Pereira et al., 2014), possibly because falls occur less often (i.e., the chance of injury is reduced), and/or the resistance to fall impact may be higher (Rose, 2008). Physical activity induces a good body composition (Rose, 2008), increasing self-resistance to injuries by reinforcing locomotion structures, namely bone and muscle (Kontulainen et al., 2004; Ross et al., 2008; Stewart et al., 2005). Different exercise programs showed to prevent fall-related injuries either by avoiding falls occurrence (the interaction between the agent and the host) or by decreasing the host susceptibility to the agent. For example, dance (Cruz-Ferreira et al., 2015; McKinley et al., 2008), water-based exercise (Devereux, Robertson, & Briffa, 2005), tai chi (Voukelatos, Cumming, Lord, & Rissel, 2007) and Pilates method programs (Irez, Ozdemir, Evin, Irez, & Korkusuz, 2011; Siqueira Rodrigues, Ali Cader, Bento Torres, Oliveira, & Martin Dantas, 2010) showed to improve physical fitness (including balance) which resulted in a decreased propensity to fall; while whole body vibration showed to improve bone mineral density (Bogaerts et al., 2011; Gusi, Raimundo, & Leal, 2006).

2.4. MAINTENANCE OF INDEPENDENCE IN OLDER ADULTS

Associated with falls, there is also a problem of independence in the accomplishment of everyday tasks that enables older adults to lead an autonomous life. Falls and fall-related injuries have been reported as a major factor restricting independence, becoming the main reason for the institutionalization of older adults (Nitz & Choy, 2008; Scheffer, Schuurmans, van Dijk, van der Hooft, & de Rooij, 2008). This undesired effect comes from physical consequences of fall-related injuries, especially fractures, which restrict the ability to perform daily tasks and are responsible for further falls (Arfken, Lach, Birge, & Miller, 1994; Denkinger et al., 2015; Donald & Bulpitt, 1999; Lloyd et al., 2009; Tinetti et al., 1994). Besides the obvious limitation created by the injury, there is a close relationship between the occurrence of fall-related injuries and a poor physical fitness that, by itself, is related with the inability to perform activities of daily living (Demura, Yamada, & Kasuga, 2012; Motl & McAuley, 2010; Rogers, Rogers, Takeshima et al., 2003). In fact, age, health status, physical activity, physical fitness, and body composition, are considered the main causes of the three outcomes analysed on the proposed theoretical model: falls, fall-related injuries, and loss of independence (Brach & VanSwearingen, 2002; Chodzko-Zajko et al., 2009; Hardy & Gill, 2005; Jung et al., 2006; Larrieu et al., 2004; Paterson & Warburton, 2010; Pluijm et al., 2006; Rikli & Jones, 2001; Sherrington et al., 2008; Stessman et al., 2005). Several studies (Aoyama et al., 2011; Kelsey et al., 2010; Pereira, 2011) reported an inverse relationship between the number of fall-related injuries and independence, which is determined by factors that affect both injuries and independence. Balance has been pointed out as the main physical parameter that explains falls occurrence. However, lower strength and gait are not least important because they not only explain the occurrence of falls but also determine independence, especially in frailer older adults (Pereira, 2011).

In addition to physical consequences of fall-related injuries, as previously mentioned, fear of falling may constitute the main reason why older adults do not carry out everyday tasks independently, even if there is no physical impairment (Cumming, Salkeld, Thomas, & Szonyi, 2000; Murphy & Tickle-Degnen, 2001). In fact, fear of falling is reported as a main psychological consequence of falls, restricting activities of daily living and, therefore, resulting in loss of independence (Landrot et al., 2007; Tinetti, Mendes de Leon, Doucette, & Baker, 1994). There are few in-depth studies on how physical activities interacts with the fear of falling and the consequent refusal to accomplish everyday tasks. Pereira and collaborators (Pereira, 2011) concluded that the people with greatest fear of falling perform less physical activity, especially vigorous physical activity, and avoid some riskier everyday tasks, such as going up and down stairs or getting objects from closets, which may lead to fewer falls and injuries. However, fear of falling is also the cause for the subject to avoid not only the riskier activities of daily living, but also activities that could be performed safely (Tinetti, Richman, & Powell, 1990). Fear of falling has been pointed as a risk factor for falls (Pluijm et al., 2006); however, Pereira and collaborators (Pereira et al., 2014) suggested that fear of falling works most as a self-perceived risk of falling due to frailty and previous experience of falling and injury (a protective mechanism) and less as a real risk factor for falling and consequent injury. Despite everything, at long term, fear of falling was pointed as a greater restrictor of the performance of activities of daily living than falls did, with or without severe injuries (Pereira, 2011). These results emphasize the importance of self-confidence in the maintenance of independence in activities of daily living that may be improved by the performance of functional exercises that mimic everyday life tasks (Pereira, 2011).

Conclusion and Recommendations

This work analyzed the factors involved in falls and their consequences. The most obvious are injuries, and the less evident, but perhaps more serious, are the fear of falling and the loss of independence. Through this analysis, we determined which and how the components described in theoretical approach (task, subject [older adult], environment; and injury agent) may be controlled in order to counteract the trend towards the rupture that will result in these undesirable events.

Our research indicates that the key components causing a rupture of the system (occurrence of falls and fall-related injuries, fear of falling, and loss of independence) in old age, considering the normal circumstances of daily living, are conditions of frailty associated with the subject. It was also noted that, as the subject becomes more fragile (that is as there is an increase the risk of intrinsic factors), their susceptibility to extrinsic risk factors rises, especially regarding the environmental hazards, as well as their difficulty in successfully meeting the demands of tasks (without falls, injuries, fear of falling or disability). Furthermore, performance of activities of daily living is restricted due to lack of self-confidence. However, a good level of physical fitness can also increase the risk of falls and fall-related injuries because the fitter people show more self-confidence in performing more demanding tasks, and in more hazardous environments, thereby exposing themselves to more dangerous situations. In fact, older adults are often not aware of their real predisposition to falls and injuries, and only identify the inherent risk of these events after the occurrence of the fall, the injury or the disability.

There is an inverse relationship between the number of fall-related injuries and independence, which is determined by factors that affect both injuries and independence. Age has been pointed as a main risk factor for these two events, however it was found that age does not work as a risk factor for falls, injuries, or dependence in the absence of health conditions associated to a good physical fitness (especially balance without neglecting lower strength and gait) and body composition (especially lean body mass). On the other hand, health conditions are reported as the most important determinant for the occurrence of falls and fall-related injuries, as well as are pointed as the most reliable indicator for explaining the fear of falling and the loss of independence. On another hand, fear of falling has been shown to be a more important explanation for the loss of independence than falls and severe injuries. People with greater fear of falling avoid some riskier tasks, which may lead to fewer falls and injuries. However, fear of falling is a determinant cause for avoiding not only the riskier activities/tasks but also activities/tasks of daily living, which could be performed safely. Thus, effective interventions to prevent loss of independence must improve older adults' self-confidence.

Physical activity has confirmed to be an effective strategy to prevent falls and consequent injuries. Probably it is because physical activity is positively associated with the ability for successfully performing tasks and also with the capacity for avoiding collision in the case of a fall (avoiding the interaction between the host and the injury agent). Physical activity decreases the negative effects of illnesses, improves physical fitness and induces a good body composition, increasing self-resistance to injuries by reinforcing locomotion structures, namely bone and muscle. However, practicing vigorous physical activity, especially in less controlled and more hazardous environments, may increase falls and fall-related injuries by increasing the exposure to dangerous situations. A balance must be found between the potential positive and negative effects of physical activity. The accumulation of at least 1,150 MET-min.wk^{-1} of physical activity, maintaining vigorous-intensity activity expenditure below 500 MET-min.wk^{-1}, seems to prevent falls and fall-related injuries.

Women are more likely to fall than men. The higher susceptibility to falls and disability in women as compared with men seems to be caused by poorer health, body composition, and physical fitness. Nevertheless, under similar conditions of health body composition and physical fitness (mainly balance), the probability of falling in men becomes higher than in women (due to the fact that men classically expose themselves to more hazardous situations).

This research was centered in independent community dwelling older adults. Thereby, some adjustment may be needed in order to generate the outcomes to very frail people, especially in case of cognitive impairments. Notwithstanding, current research outlaw the follow primary recommendations for fall and fall-related injuries prevention:

- A healthy lifestyle, in order to avoid co-morbidities or, at least, to minimize its effects.
- The reduction of environmental hazards, principally when fitness decreases and frailty increases, and the restraint of difficult tasks in hazardous environments.
- The practice at least 1,150 MET-min.wk^{-1} of physical activity, with no more than 500 MET-min.wk^{-1} (~60 min. wk^{-1}) of vigorous physical activity (due to associated hazards). For example a combination of 1 hour of walking, 2 hours of moderate physical activity (such as carrying light loads or bicycling at a regular pace) and 20 minutes of vigorous physical activity (such as heavy lifting, digging, aerobics, or fast bicycling) per week, what computes ~1,150 MET-min.wk^{-1}.
- The implementation of exercise programs to prevent physical fitness loss, especially balance. Further, muscle strength and gait exercises may be particularly relevant for less fit and frail people.
- The performance of functional exercises that mimic everyday life tasks and promote self-confidence.
- Regarding women, special attention must be taken because they tend to be more fragile. Regarding men, special attention must be taken because they tend to expose themselves to more hazardous situations.

References

Achour, E., Barthelemy, J., Lionard, K., Trombert, B., Lacour, J., Thomas-Anterion, C. (2011). Level of physical activity at the age of 65 predicts successful aging seven years later: the PROOF study. *Rejuvenation Res, 14*(2), 215-221.

Alamgir, H., Muazzam, S., & Nasrullah, M. (2012). Unintentional falls mortality among elderly in the United States: Time for action. *Injury, 43*(12), 2065-2071.

Ambrose, A., Paul, G., & Hausdorff, J. (2013). Risk factors for falls among older adults: a review of the literature. *Maturitas, 75*(1), 51-61.

Aoyama, M., Suzuki, Y., Onishi, J., & Kuzuya, M. (2011). Physical and functional factors in activities of daily living that predict falls in community-dwelling older women. *Geriatr Gerontol Int, 11*(3), 348-357.

Arfken, C. L., Lach, H. W., Birge, S. J., & Miller, J. P. (1994). The prevalence and correlates of fear of falling in elderly persons living in the community. *Am J Public Health, 84*(4), 565-570.

Association of Emergency Medical Technicians, A. C. o. S. (2003). Injury Prevention (C. 1, Trans.) *PHTLS, Basic and Advanced Prehospital Trauma Life Support.* (5 ed., pp. 10-25). St. Louis, Missouri: Mosby.

Barrett-Connor, E., Weiss, T., McHorney, C., Miller, P., & Siris, E. (2009). Predictors of falls among postmenopausal women: results from the National Osteoporosis Risk Assessment (NORA). *Osteoporos Int, 20*(5), 715-722.

Bateni, H., Zecevic, A., MacIlroy, W., & Maki, E. (2004). Resolving conflicts in task demands during balance recovery: does holding an object inhibit compensatory grasping? *Exp Brain Res, 157*, 49-58.

Bath, P., & Morgan, K. (1999). Differential risk profiles for indoor and outdoor falls in older people living in home in Nottingham, UK. *Eur J Epidemiol, 15*, 65-73.

Bialoszewski, D., Slupik, A., Lewczuk, E., Gotlib, J., Mosiolek, A., & Mierzwinska, A. (2008). Incidence of falls and their effect on mobility of individuals over 65 years of age relative to their place of residence. *Ortop Traumatol Rehabil, 10*(5), 441-448.

Bogaerts, A., Delecluse, C., Boonen, S., Claessens, A. L., Milisen, K., & Verschueren, S. M. (2011). Changes in balance, functional performance and fall risk following whole body vibration training and vitamin D supplementation in institutionalized elderly women. A 6 month randomized controlled trial. *Gait Posture, 33*(3), 466-472.

Brach, J., & VanSwearingen, J. (2002). Physical impairment and disability: relationship to performance of activities of daily living in community-dwelling older men. *Phys Ther, 82*(8), 752-761.

Braun, B. (1998). Knowledge and perception of fall-related risk factors and fall-reduction techniques among community-dwelling elderly individuals. *Phys Ther, 78*(12), 1262-1276.

Britton, A., Shipley, M., Singh-Manoux, A., & Marmot, M. G. (2008). Successful aging: the contribution of early-life and midlife risk factors. *J Am Geriatr Soc, 56*(6), 1098-1105.

Brown, J., & Josse, R. (2002). 2002 clinical practice guidelines for the diagnosis and management of osteoporosis in Canada. *CMAJ, 12*(167), S1-S34.

Cadarette, S., Jaglal, S., Kreiger, N., McIsaac, W., Darlington, G., & Tu, J. (2000). Development and validation of the Osteoporosis Risk Assessment Instrument to facilitate selection of women for bone densitometry. *CMAJ, 162*(9), 1289-1294.

Carter, N. D., Khan, K. M., McKay, H. A., Petit, M. A., Waterman, C., Heinonen, A. (2002). Community-based exercise program reduces risk factors for falls in 65- to 75-year-old women with osteoporosis: randomised controlled trial. *CMAJ, 167*(9), 997-1004.

Chan, B. K., Marshall, L. M., Winters, K. M., Faulkner, K. A., Schwartz, A. V., & Orwoll, E. S. (2007). Incident fall risk and physical activity and physical performance among older men: the Osteoporotic Fractures in Men Study. *Am J Epidemiol, 165*(6), 696-703.

Chodzko-Zajko, W., Proctor, D., Fiatarone Singh, M., Minson, C., Nigg, C., Salem, G. (2009). American College of Sports Medicine position stand. Exercise and physical activity for older adults. *Med Sci Sports Exerc, 41*(7), 1510-1530.

Chu, L., Chi, I., & Chiu, A. (2005). Incidence and predictors of falls in the chinese elderly. *Ann Acad Med Singapore, 34*(1), 60-72.

Cooper, J. W., & Burfield, A. H. (2009). Medication interventions for fall prevention in the older adult. *J Am Pharm Assoc (2003), 49*(3), e70-82; quiz e83-74.

Cornillon, E., Blanchon, M., Ramboatsisetraina, P., Braize, C., Beauchet, V., Dubost, V. (2002). Impact d`un programme de prévention multidisciplinaire de la chute chez le sujet âgé autonome vivant à domicile, avec analyse avant-après des performances physiques. *Ann Phys Rehabil Med, 45*(9), 493-504.

Coutinho, E. S., Fletcher, A., Bloch, K. V., & Rodrigues, L. C. (2008). Risk factors for falls with severe fracture in elderly people living in a middle-income country: a case control study. *BMC Geriatr, 8*, 21.

Crimmins, E. M., Hayward, M. D., Hagedorn, A., Saito, Y., & Brouard, N. (2009). Change in disability-free life expectancy for Americans 70-years-old and older. *Demography, 46*(3), 627-646.

Cruz-Ferreira, A., Marmeleira, J., Formigo, A., Gomes, D., & Fernandes, J. (2015). Creative Dance Improves Physical Fitness and Life Satisfaction in Older Women. *Res Aging*, 1-19.

Cumming, R. G., Salkeld, G., Thomas, M., & Szonyi, G. (2000). Prospective study of the impact of fear of falling on activities of daily living, SF-36 scores, and nursing home admission. *J Gerontol A Biol Sci Med Sci, 55*(5), M299-305.

Davids, K., Glazier, P., Araujo, D., & Bartlett, R. (2003). Movement systems as dynamical systems: the functional role of variability and its implications for sports medicine. *Sports Med, 33*(4), 245-260.

de Rekeneire, N., Visser, M., Peila, R., Nevitt, M., Cauley, J., Tylavsky, F. (2003). Is a fall just a fall: correlates of falling in healthy older persons. The Health, Aging and Body Composition Study. *J Am Geriatr Soc, 51*(6), 841-846.

Demura, S., Yamada, T., & Kasuga, K. (2012). Severity of injuries associated with falls in the community dwelling elderly are not affected by fall characteristics and physical function level. *Arch Gerontol Geriatr, 55*(1), 186-189.

Denkinger, M., Lukas, A., Nikolaus, T., & Hauer, K. (2015). Factors associated with fear of falling and associated activity restriction in community-dwelling older adults: a systematic review. *Am J Geriatr Psychiatry, 23*(1), 72-86.

Devereux, K., Robertson, D., & Briffa, N. K. (2005). Effects of a water-based program on women 65 years and over: a randomised controlled trial. *Aust J Physiother, 51*(2), 102-108.

Donald, I. P., & Bulpitt, C. J. (1999). The prognosis of falls in elderly people living at home. *Age Ageing, 28*(2), 121-125.

Douglas, A. Y., Mehan, T. J., Collins, C. L., Smith, G. A., & McKenzie, L. B. (2009). Acute computer-related injuries treated in U.S. emergency departments, 1994-2006. *Am J Prev Med, 37*(1), 24-28.

Etman, A., Wijlhuizen, G., van Heuvelen, M., Chorus, A., & Hopman-Rock, M. (2012). Falls incidence underestimates the risk of fall-related injuries in older age groups: a comparison with the FARE (Falls risk by Exposure). *Age Ageing, 41*(2), 190-195.

Eurostat. (2014). *Key figures on the enlargement countries* Retrieved from http://ec.europa.eu/eurostat/web/products-pocketbooks/-/KS-GM-13-001.

Fuzhong, L., Fisher, K. J., Harmer, P., MacAuley, E., & Wilson, N. L. (2003). Fear of falling in elderly persons: association with falls, functional ability and quality of life. *J Gerontol B Psychol Sci Soc Sci., 58*(5), 283-290.

Gill, D., Zou, G., Jones, G., & Speechley, M. (2008). Injurious falls are associated with lower household but higher recreational physical activities in community-dwelling older male veterans. *Gerontology, 54*(2), 106-115.

Gill, T. M., Gahbauer, E. A., Lin, H., Han, L., & Allore, H. G. (2013). Comparisons between older men and women in the trajectory and burden of disability over the course of nearly 14 years. *J Am Med Dir Assoc, 14*(4), 280-286.

Gillespie, L. D., Gillespie, W. J., Robertson, M. C., Lamb, S. E., Cumming, R. G., & Rowe, B. H. (2009). WITHDRAWN: Interventions for preventing falls in elderly people. *Cochrane Database Syst Rev*(2), CD000340.

Gitlin, L. N., Winter, L., Dennis, M. P., Corcoran, M., Schinfeld, S., & Hauck, W. W. (2006). A randomized trial of a multicomponent home intervention to reduce functional difficulties in older adults. *J Am Geriatr Soc, 54*(5), 809-816.

Glazier, P. S., & Davids, K. (2009). Constraints on the complete optimization of human motion. *Sports Med, 39*(1), 15-28.

Goldacre, M. J., Roberts, S. E., & Yeates, D. (2002). Mortality after admission to hospital with fractured neck of femur: database study. *BMJ, 325*(7369), 868-869.

Gregg, E. W., Cauley, J. A., Seeley, D. G., Ensrud, K. E., & Bauer, D. C. (1998). Physical activity and osteoporotic fracture risk in older women. Study of Osteoporotic Fractures Research Group. *Ann Intern Med, 129*(2), 81-88.

Gusi, N., Raimundo, A., & Leal, A. (2006). Low-frequency vibratory exercise reduces the risk of bone fracture more than walking: a randomized controlled trial. *BMC Musculoskelet Disord, 7*, 92.

Hardy, S. E., & Gill, T. M. (2005). Factors associated with recovery of independence among newly disabled older persons. *Arch Intern Med, 165*(1), 106-112.

Hashimoto, S., Kawado, M., Seko, R., Murakami, Y., Hayashi, M., Kato, M. (2010). Trends in disability-free life expectancy in Japan, 1995-2004. *J Epidemiol, 20*(4), 308-312.

Hogan, D. B., MacDonald, F. A., Betts, J., Bricker, S., Ebly, E. M., Delarue, B. (2001). A randomized controlled trial of a community-based consultation service to prevent falls. *CMAJ, 165*(5), 537-543.

Hundrup, Y. A., Ekholm, O., Hoidrup, S., Davidsen, M., & Obel, E. B. (2005). Risk factors for hip fracture and a possible effect modification by hormone replacement therapy. The Danish nurse cohort study. *Eur J Epidemiol, 20*(10), 871-877.

INE;IP. (2009). Projections of Resident Population - Portugal - 2008 - 2060. Retrieved from: http://www.ine.pt

Irez, G. B., Ozdemir, R. A., Evin, R., Irez, S. G., & Korkusuz, F. (2011). Integrating pilates exercise into an exercise program for 65+ year-old women to reduce falls. *J Sports Sci Med, 10*(1), 105-111.

Jung, S. H., Ostbye, T., & Park, K. O. (2006). A longitudinal study of the relationship between health behavior risk factors and dependence in activities of daily living. *J Prev Med Public Health, 39*(3), 221-228.

Kanis, J. (2002). Osteoporosis III: diagnostic of osteoporosis and assessment of fracture risk. *Lancet, 359*(9321), 1929-1936.

Kannus, P. (2006). How to prevent fractures due to accidental falls among elderly population. *Duodecim, 122*(2), 135-137.

Kannus, P., Sievanen, H., Palvanen, M., Jarvinen, T., & Parkkari, J. (2005). Prevention of falls and consequent injuries in elderly people. *Lancet, 366*(9500), 1885-1893.

Karinkanta, S., Heinonen, A., Sievanen, H., Uusi-Rasi, K., Fogelholm, M., & Kannus, P. (2009). Maintenance of exercise-induced benefits in physical functioning and bone among elderly women. *Osteoporos Int, 20*(4), 665-674.

Kelsey, J. L., Berry, S. D., Procter-Gray, E., Quach, L., Nguyen, U. S., Li, W. (2010). Indoor and outdoor falls in older adults are different: the maintenance of balance, independent living, intellect, and Zest in the Elderly of Boston Study. *J Am Geriatr Soc, 58*(11), 2135-2141.

Kontulainen, S., Heinonen, A., Kannus, P., Pasanen, M., Sievanen, H., & Vuori, I. (2004). Former exercisers of an 18-month intervention display residual a BMD benefits compared with control women 3,5 years post-intervention: a follow-up of a randomised controlled high-impact trial. *Osteoporos Int, 15*.

Laing, A. C., & Robinovitch, S. N. (2009). Low stiffness floors can attenuate fall-related femoral impact forces by up to 50% without substantially impairing balance in older women. *Accid Anal Prev, 41*(3), 642-650.

Lamontagne, I., Levesque, B., Gingras, S., Maurice, P., & Verreault, R. (2004). Environmental hazards for falls in elders in low income housing. *Rev Epidemiol Sante Publique, 52*(1), 19-27.

Landrot M, R., Perrot, C., Blanc, P., Beauchet, O., Blanchon, M. A., & Gonthier, R. (2007). Does the care for the fear of falling bring a profit to community living elderly people who had experienced falls? *Psychol Neuropsychiatr Vieil, 5*(3), 225-234.

Larrieu, S., Peres, K., Letenneur, L., Berr, C., Dartigues, J. F., Ritchie, K. (2004). Relationship between body mass index and different domains of disability in older persons: the 3C study. *Int J Obes Relat Metab Disord, 28*(12), 1555-1560.

Lenze, E. J., Munin, M. C., Skidmore, E. R., Amanda Dew, M., Rogers, J. C., Whyte, E. M. (2007). Onset of depression in elderly persons after hip fracture: implications for prevention and early intervention of late-life depression. *J Am Geriatr Soc, 55*(1), 81-86.

Li, W., Keegan, T. H., Sternfeld, B., Sidney, S., Quesenberry, C. P., Jr., & Kelsey, J. L. (2006). Outdoor falls among middle-aged and older adults: a neglected public health problem. *Am J Public Health, 96*(7), 1192-1200.

Liu-Ambrose, T., Kan, K., Eng, J., Gillies, G., Lord, R., & McKay, H. (2005). The beneficial effects of group-based exercises on fall risk profile and physical activity persist 1 year postintervention in older women with low bone mass: follow-up after withdrawal of exercise. *J Am Geriatr Soc, 53*, 1767-1773.

Lloyd, B. D., Williamson, D. A., Singh, N. A., Hansen, R. D., Diamond, T. H., Finnegan, T. P. (2009). Recurrent and injurious falls in the year following hip fracture: a prospective study of incidence and risk factors from the Sarcopenia and Hip Fracture study. *J Gerontol A Biol Sci Med Sci, 64*(5), 599-609.

Marmeleira, J. F., Pereira, C., Cruz-Ferreira, A., Fretes, V., Pisco, R., & Fernandes, O. M. (2009). Creative dance can enhance proprioception in older adults. *J Sports Med Phys Fitness, 49*(4), 480-485.

McKinley, P., Jacobson, A., Leroux, A., Bednarczyk, V., Rossignol, M., & Fung, J. (2008). Effect of a community-based Argentine tango dance program on functional balance and confidence in older adults. *J Aging Phys Act, 16*(4), 435-453.

McLean, K., Day, L., & Dalton, A. Economic evaluation of a group-based exercise program for falls prevention among the older community-dwelling population. *BMC Geriatr, 15*, 33.

Menant, J. C., Steele, J. R., Menz, H. B., Munro, B. J., & Lord, S. R. (2008). Optimizing footwear for older people at risk of falls. *J Rehabil Res Dev, 45*(8), 1167-1181.

Minino, A. M., Heron, M. P., Murphy, S. L., & Kochanek, K. D. (2007). Deaths: final data for 2004. *Natl Vital Stat Rep, 55*(19), 1-119.

Motl, R. W., & McAuley, E. (2010). Physical activity, disability, and quality of life in older adults. *Phys Med Rehabil Clin N Am, 21*(2), 299-308.

Murphy, S., & Tickle-Degnen, L. (2001). Participation in daily living tasks among older adults with fear of falling. *Am J Occup Ther, 55*(5), 538-544.

Nelson, M. E., Rejeski, W. J., Blair, S. N., Duncan, P. W., Judge, J. O., King, A. C. (2007). Physical activity and public health in older adults: recommendation from the American College of Sports Medicine and the American Heart Association. *Circulation, 116*(9), 1094-1105.

Nitz, J. C., & Choy, N. L. (2008). Falling is not just for older women: support for pre-emptive prevention intervention before 60. *Climacteric, 11*(6), 461-466.

Nosraty, L., Jylha, M., Raittila, T., & Lumme-Sandt, K. (2015). Perceptions by the oldest old of successful aging, Vitality 90+ Study. *J Aging Stud, 32*, 50-58.

Nyman, S. R., & Victor, C. R. (2012). Older people's participation in and engagement with falls prevention interventions in community settings: an augment to the Cochrane systematic review. *Age Ageing, 41*(1), 16-23.

Ojha, H. A., Kern, R. W., Lin, C. H., & Winstein, C. J. (2009). Age affects the attentional demands of stair ambulation: evidence from a dual-task approach. *Phys Ther, 89*(10), 1080-1088.

Ojo, P., O'Connor, J., Kim, D., Ciardiello, K., & Bonadies, J. (2009). Patterns of injury in geriatric falls. *Conn Med, 73*(3), 139-145.

Oliver, D., Britton, M., Seed, P., Martin, F., & Hopper, A. (1997). Development and evaluation of evidence based risk assessment tool (stratify) to predict which elderly inpatients will fall: Case-control and cohort studies. *BMJ, 315*, 1049-1053.

Paterson, D. H., & Warburton, D. E. (2010). Physical activity and functional limitations in older adults: a systematic review related to Canada's Physical Activity Guidelines. *Int J Behav Nutr Phys Act, 7*, 38.

Peeters, G. M., Verweij, L. M., van Schoor, N. M., Pijnappels, M., Pluijm, S. M., Visser, M. (2010). Which types of activities are associated with risk of recurrent falling in older persons? *J Gerontol A Biol Sci Med Sci, 65*(7), 743-750.

Pereira, C. (2011). *Risk of Falls, Fear of Falling, and Loss of Autonomy on Old Women: Impact of Physical Activity and Fitness in the Performance of Activities of Daily Living.* (PhD), Faculdade de Motricidade Humana, Universidade Técnica de Lisboa, Lisbon.

Pereira, C., & Baptista, F. (2012). Variation of the different attributes that support the physical function in community-dwelling older adults. *J Sports Med Phys Fitness, 52*(2), 190-197.

Pereira, C., Baptista, F., & Infante, P. (2013). Men Older than 50 Yrs Are More Likely to Fall than Women Under Similar Conditions of Health, Body Composition, and Balance. *Am J Phys Med Rehabil, 92*(12), 1095-1103.

Pereira, C., Baptista, F., & Infante, P. (2014). Role of physical activity in the occurrence of falls and fall-related injuries in community-dwelling adults over 50 years old. *Disabil Rehabil, 36*(2), 117-124.

Pereira, C., Vogelaere, P., & Baptista, F. (2008). Role of physical activity in the prevention of falls and their consequences in the elderly. *Eur Rev Aging Phys Act, 5*(1), 51-58.

Pluijm, S. (2001). *Predictors and consequences of falls and fractures in the elderly.* Vrije Universiteit, Amesterdam.

Pluijm, S., Smit, J., Tromp, E., Stel, V., Deeg, D., Bouter, L. M. (2006). A risk profile for identifying community-dwelling elderly with a high risk of recurrent falling: results of a 3-year prospective study. *Osteoporos Int, 17*(3), 417-425.

Pynnonen, K., Tormakangas, T., Heikkinen, R. L., Rantanen, T., & Lyyra, T. M. (2012). Does social activity decrease risk for institutionalization and mortality in older people? *J Gerontol B Psychol Sci Soc Sci, 67*(6), 765-774.

Reuben, D., & Solomon, D. (1989). Assessment in geriatrics. Of caveats and names. *J Am Geriatr Soc, 37*(6), 570-572.

Rikli, R., & Jones, C. J. (1999). Functional fitness normative scores for community-residing older adults. *J Aging Phys Act, 7*, 160-179.

Rikli, R., & Jones, J. (2001). *Senior Fitness Test Manual.* Champaign, Ilinois, USA: Human Kinetics.

Robbins, J. A., Biggs, M. L., & Cauley, J. (2006). Adjusted mortality after hip fracture: From the cardiovascular health study. *J Am Geriatr Soc, 54*(12), 1885-1891.

Rogers, M., Rogers, N., Chaparro, B., Stumpfhauser, L., & Halcomb, C. (2003). Effects of modular course training on mobility in older adults aged 79-90 years. *Disabil Rehabil, 25*(4-5), 213-217.

Rogers, M., Rogers, N., Takeshima, N., & Islam, M. (2003). Methods to assess and improve the physical parameters associated with fall risk in older adults. *Prev Med, 36*(3), 255-264.

Rose, D. J. (2008). Preventing falls among older adults: no "one size suits all" intervention strategy. *J Rehabil Res Dev, 45*(8), 1153-1166.

Ross, R., Berentzen, T., Bradshaw, A. J., Janssen, I., Kahn, H. S., Katzmarzyk, P. T. (2008). Does the relationship between waist circumference, morbidity and mortality depend on measurement protocol for waist circumference? *Obes Rev, 9*(4), 312-325.

Scheffer, A. C., Schuurmans, M. J., van Dijk, N., van der Hooft, T., & de Rooij, S. E. (2008). Fear of falling: measurement strategy, prevalence, risk factors and consequences among older persons. *Age Ageing, 37*(1), 19-24.

Sherrington, C., Whitney, J. C., Lord, S. R., Herbert, R. D., Cumming, R. G., & Close, J. C. (2008). Effective exercise for the prevention of falls: a systematic review and meta-analysis. *J Am Geriatr Soc, 56*(12), 2234-2243.

Siqueira Rodrigues, B. G., Ali Cader, S., Bento Torres, N. V., Oliveira, E. M., & Martin Dantas, E. H. (2010). Pilates method in personal autonomy, static balance and quality of life of elderly females. *J Bodyw Mov Ther, 14*(2), 195-202.

Spector, W. D., & Fleishman, J. A. (1998). Combining activities of daily living with instrumental activities of daily living to measure functional disability. *J Gerontol B Psychol Sci Soc Sci, 53*(1), S46-57.

Stessman, J., Hammerman-Rozenberg, R., Maaravi, Y., Azoulai, D., & Cohen, A. (2005). Strategies to enhance longevity and independent function: the Jerusalem Longitudinal Study. *Mech Ageing Dev, 126*(2), 327-331.

Stevens, J. A., Thomas, K., Teh, L., & Greenspan, A. I. (2009). Unintentional Fall Injuries Associated with Walkers and Canes in Older Adults Treated in U.S. Emergency Departments. *J Am Geriatr Soc,* 57(8):1464-9.

Stewart, K., Bacher, A., Hees, P., Tayback, M., Ouyang, P., & Beur, S. (2005). Exercise effects on bone mineral density. Relationships to change in fitness and fatness. *Am J Prev Med, 28*(5), 453-460.

Tak, E., Kuiper, R., Chorus, A., & Hopman-Rock, M. (2014). Prevention of onset and progression of basic ADL disability by physical activity in community dwelling older adults: a meta-analysis. *Ageing Res Rev, 12*(1), 329-338.

Tinetti, M. (2003). Preventing falls in elderly persons. *N Engl J Med, 348*(1), 42-49.

Tinetti, M., Baker, D., MacAvay, G., Claus, E., Garrett, P., Gottschalk, M. (1994). A multifactorial intervention to reduce the risk of falling among elderly people living in the community. *N Engl J Med, 331*(13), 821-827.

Tinetti, M., Richman, D., & Powell, L. (1990). Falls efficacy as a measure of fear of falling. *J Gerontol, 45*(6), P239-243.

Tinetti, M., & Speechley, M. (1989). Prevention of falls among the elderly. *N Engl J Med, 320*(16), 1055-1059.

Tinetti, M., Speechley, M., & Ginter, S. (1988). Risk factor for falls among elderly living in the community. *N Engl J Med, 319*(26), 1701-1707.

Tinetti, M., Mendes de Leon, C. F., Doucette, J. T., & Baker, D. I. (1994). Fear of falling and fall-related efficacy in relationship to functioning among community-living elders. *J Gerontol, 49*(3), M140-147.

van Heuvelen, M. J., Hochstenbach, J., de Greef, M. H., Brouwer, W. H., Mulder, T., & Scherder, E. (2005). Is the Activities-specific Balance Confidence Scale suitable for Dutch older persons living in the community? *Tijdschr Gerontol Geriatr, 36*(4), 146-154.

Vasquez, E., Batsis, J. A., Germain, C. M., & Shaw, B. A. (2014). Impact of obesity and physical activity on functional outcomes in the elderly: data from NHANES 2005-2010. *J Aging Health, 26*(6), 1032-1046.

Vitetta, L., & Anton, B. (2007). Lifestyle and nutrition, caloric restriction, mitochondrial health and hormones: scientific interventions for anti-aging. *Clin Interv Aging, 2*(4), 537-543.

Voukelatos, A., Cumming, R. G., Lord, S. R., & Rissel, C. (2007). A randomized, controlled trial of tai chi for the prevention of falls: the Central Sydney tai chi trial. *J Am Geriatr Soc, 55*(8), 1185-1191.

Vouriot, A., Gauchard, G., Chau, N., Benamghar, L., Lepori, M., Mur, J. (2004). Sensorial organization favoring higher visual contributions is a risk facto of falls in an occupational. *Neurosci Res, 48*(3), 239-247.

Wang, X., Li, X., Shen, X., & Agrawal, C. M. (2003). Age-related changes of noncalcified collagen in human cortical bone. *Ann Biomed Eng, 31*(11), 1365-1371.

WHO. (2010). World Health Statistics 2010. Retrieved 28 December 2010, from http://www.who.int/whosis/whostat/2010/en/index.html

Wijlhuizen, G. J., Chorus, A. M., & Hopman-Rock, M. (2010). The FARE: a new way to express FAlls Risk among older persons including physical activity as a measure of exposure. *Prev Med, 50*(3), 143-147.

Yeo, Y. Y., Lee, S. K., Lim, C. Y., Quek, L. S., & Ooi, S. B. (2009). A review of elderly injuries seen in a Singapore emergency department. *Singapore Med J, 50*(3), 278-283.

Yokoya, T., Demura, S., & Sato, S. (2009). Three-year follow-up of the fall risk and physical function characteristics of the elderly participating in a community exercise class. *J Physiol Anthropol, 28*(2), 55-62.

Zijlstra, G., Haastregt, J., Eijk, J., & Kempen, G. (2005). Evaluating an intervention to reduce fear o falling and associated activity restriction in elderly persons: design of a randomised controlled trial. *BMC Public Health, 5*(26), 1-9.

In: Accidental Falls
Editor: Brenda Evans
ISBN: 978-1-63483-228-1

Chapter 3

FALL PREVENTION IN A PERSON WITH PARKINSON'S DISEASE: A CASE STUDY REPORT

Lynne M. Chapman, MS, OTR/L, LICDC
Clinical Assistant Professor/Coordinator of Professional Development/Senior Clinician
Department of Occupational Therapy
The University of Toledo, Toledo, OH, US

ABSTRACT

A sensorimotor approach that included the use of repetitive, fast, and gross movement patterns was chosen for as the theoretical foundation for this case study. This approach is intended for use across disciplines and the principles of this approach have been correlated with fall prevention in persons who have a diagnosis of Parkinson's disease. It was hypothesized that there would be a significant decrease in the reported number of falls following successful completion of intervention that consisted of the use of the sensorimotor approach to intervention. The intervention included preparatory, purposeful, and occupation-based interventions using fast, repetitive gross motor patterns of movement. The goal of this sensorimotor approach was to teach the participant a new way of moving that would now be required in order to safety engage in everyday occupations. The process of learning and using new ways of moving by altering the effort required and type of movement required for task completion is a phenomenon referred to in the literature as "recalibration." Upon completion of the intervention, the participant had achieved success in gaining a new awareness of the effort required to internally regulate the movements required for safe and successful completion of occupations of daily living. The average rate of reported falls prior to the participant's participation in the study was one per month and at six month follow-up from the initiation of his participation in the study, patient had no falls to report.

Keywords: Parkinson's disease, fall prevention, sensorimotor approach

Background Information

This case study describes the evaluation and intervention process utilized with a participant in a small randomized trial entitled, Multicomponent home-based therapy in Parkinson's. The participant described in this case was randomly assigned to the intervention group which consisted of an in-home occupational therapy evaluation and intervention, to include his community. The goal of the intervention was to increase the participant's ability to engage in everyday occupations that had personal meaning to him. The occupational therapist and the participant worked collaboratively to find ways of improving the participant's safety, especially his risk of falls given the fact that he had reported a total number of 12 falls within the year prior to the initiation of his participation in this study.

The participant described in this case is a 78-year-old male with a diagnosis of Parkinson's disease. He was born and raised in the same town where he currently resides. He lives with his spouse who is employed full-time. On weekdays, the participant is home alone while his spouse is at work. The participant lives in a one story home with no steps to enter. His bathroom is equipped with a tub and shower combined. The participant had reported twelve falls within the past year. He stated that he had never having had a home safety evaluation by an occupational therapist.

The medications specific to the treatment of his Parkinson's symptoms at the time of the intervention included Sinemat Reg (24/100, 1½), Sinemat CR (50/100 QID), Aricept (10 to make some changes to his home, as well as to teach and practice new ways of doing some occupations. mg qd), and Persantine (50 mg, tid). Co-morbidities included congestive heart failure, hypertension, hypercholesteremia, and a history of a coronary artery bypass graft. Current medications for these co-morbidities included Coumadin, Lasix, Kloreform, Levothyvoxin, and Simvastatin.

IDENTIFIED NEED

Parkinson's disease (PD) is the second most common neurodegenerative disease, after Alzheimer's disease. With a mean age of diagnosis at 62 years, approximately 1.6% of the people 65 years and older suffer from PD, and incidence and prevalence increase with age. Most of the 1.5 million Americans with PD have significant impairments in speech and movement that negatively impact their quality of life. As the number of elderly older than 65 years increases, the prevalence of PD is predicted to grow four-fold by 2040.

For the 60,000 individuals diagnosed annually with PD, therapeutic options that modify disease progression are needed. The goals of rehabilitation for persons with PD typically include improved cardiovascular fitness, strength, range of motion, posture, gait, coordination, and balance. Strategies that are specific to this population that are commonly utilized include auditory, visual, and tactile cueing to improve mobility and to overcome freezing. The use of simplistic occupations and environmental modifications are interventions commonly utilized by occupational therapists working with persons with PD as compensations, based upon the premise that neurophysiologic improvement is not feasible.

THEORETICAL APPROACH

A sensorimotor approach to intervention was chosen for this study because the foundational principles are based upon the premise that repeated, rapid, gross motor movements provide the kinesthetic feedback required in order that persons with PD learn the amount of excursion and the type of movements that will allow them to successfully participate in occupations of daily living. This process or "recalibration" of movements has been associated with a reduction in falls in persons with PD. These movement patterns can be utilized as preparatory, purposeful, or occupation-based.

A sensorimotor approach to intervention suggests that patterns of movement are interdependent and that repetition improves the quality of movements. Protective responses to movement during engagement in occupation are often delayed or absent in persons who have PD due to the inability to initiate quick movements that require contraction of the agonist muscle and relaxation of the antagonist muscles. In persons with PD, basic movement patterns are no longer reflexive.

Persons with PD have difficulty maintaining co-contraction of tonic/static muscles, a pre-requisite for both proximal and distal joint stability. As a result, "holding" positions that require a simultaneous contraction of the agonist & antagonist are difficult for persons with PD. This ability to stabilize provides the foundation for postural control required for efficient and safe mobility.

During occupations that require heavy work, mobility is imposed on stability. The proximal joints and muscles are mobile, while the distal muscles fixate. Occupations that require lifting, carrying, pushing, and pulling require the recruitment of heavy work patterns. Occupations that require fine motor skills require stability of the proximal joints and muscles to allow for mobility of the distal joints. Factors that impact the difficulty with efficient and safe engagement in occupations for persons with PD are influenced by the degree of stability and mobility required for each specific occupation. Therefore, interventions for persons with PD must be "occupation-specific." The level of occupations performed during the intervention must be graded, based upon the required amount of proximal and distal stability specific to each occupation.

Gross motor movement patterns that require flexion provide responses that are protective. Protective responses also require quick movements of the proximal muscles. The motor patterns that facilitate these responses include rolling. Rolling should be initiated using flexion of arm & leg on same side. Rolling requires the use of the extremities and the activation of the lateral trunk muscles. Rolling stimulates the semicircular canals of the vestibular system, which activate the head and neck and ocular movements. Bed mobility that requires rolling is a prime example of the purposeful occupation that was integrated into the intervention of the participant in this case.

Neck co-contraction is a pattern of stability that precedes the control of the trunk and extremities. Maintaining the head and neck in upright against gravity requires co-contraction of the flexors & extensors of the neck and facilitates neck stability and ocular control. Persons with PD benefit from preparatory occupations provide the kinesthetic feedback required for maintaining the head and neck in upright to improve overall posture, oral motor control including swallowing and respiration required for deep breathing, phonation, and vocalization. Extension of the head and neck facilitate ocular control which is associated with improved safety with mobility since the vision is a contributing factor in balance and gait.

Sensory input can be utilized to elicit specific types and patterns of movement. Stimulation of the primary, proximal sensory systems has the tremendous potential to facilitate movement. Facilitation techniques are utilized to stimulate the reticular activating system required for alertness and muscles required to maintain upright posture. Proprioceptive stimuli from movement, activates the stretch reflexes required to achieve and maintain positions. Joint compression that requires co-contraction of muscles around joint facilitates stability to allow for mobility. Resistance is effective in facilitating movements. Vestibular input through the semicircular canals improves righting & equilibrium reactions by facilitating ocular movements. Stimulation of the utricle & saccule increase joint stability and organization required for movement. Vestibular input can be varied through movements in the axial, rotary, and diagonal planes. Directions of motion can include linear, orbital, or inversion. A fast rate stimulates movement. Rhythmical and repetitive movements elicit movement. Stimulation of the higher level, distal sensory systems that include auditory and visual input are also powerful in eliciting adaptive responses.

The sensorimotor approach to intervention requires that sensory input be immediately followed with occupation, or integrated into occupation. Using this approach, naturalistic contexts that include home and community have the potential to improve the effectiveness of the intervention by allowing for the generalization of newly learned patterns of movement to everyday occupation.

Recent scientific advances suggest that a sensorimotor approach to movement can be utilized in preparation for engagement in occupations, as well as during engagement in occupation. Studies have demonstrated that the adult brain is altered by engagement in occupation. The speed and complexity of specific occupations have been shown to be important factors in neuroplasticity. Structures of central nervous system are grouped into higher, middle & lower level structures. The middle level includes the basal ganglia. This level of brain helps to regulate and control volitional, conscious movement. In persons with PD, the basal ganglia can no longer regulate and exert control over the lower level structures. This results in a regression to primitive movement patterns.

This case study will provide the theoretical foundation for the use of a sensorimotor approach to occupations within the context of home and community. This case study will introduce the use of a sensorimotor approach during occupation in a person with a diagnosis of Parkinson's disease. This case study demonstrates how occupational therapists can integrate the principles of a sensorimotor approach in persons with PD to improve neuroplasticity through engagement in occupations of daily living in order to prevent falls. Since this approach to intervention is "occupation-specific" for people with Parkinson's disease, it is critical that persons with this condition integrate this approach into the actual engagement in occupation.

Throughout the course of the intervention, adaptive equipment that was utilized to provide sensory input through the more distal, higher level visual and auditory systems included the use of a laser cane and metronome to provide visual and auditory pacing to prevent freezing at doorways within the participant's home.

Preparatory and purposeful occupations included the practice of sustained positions as well as fast repetitions of gross motor movements in preparation for mobility and engagement in occupations of daily living. Movements that were practiced and then incorporated into the intervention included reaching from floor-to-ceiling and side-to-side; stepping and reaching forwards, sideways, and backwards; and, rocking and reaching forward. Auditory cueing was utilized to provide sensory feedback for improved quality of movements. Manual contact was utilized to improve patterns of movement through proprioceptive input that included stretching to achieve desired movements modeled by the therapist.

Initially, occupations of daily living that required less effort and consisted of simple units of movements were targeted, with a gradual progression towards occupations that required varied and complex movements and increased effort. Initially, occupations that required stabilization using postural alignment were introduced. Postural alignment was reinforced throughout all occupations of daily living. The speed and amplitude of the movements used during engagement in occupations that required reaching and transitional movements with feedback provided to improve awareness of inefficient movements and to reinforce efficient ones in an effort to improve the participant's ability to monitor his own patterns of movement. The final session included family education with the goal of teaching the participant's spouse regarding ways to provide cueing and instruction techniques for carryover of these concepts while the participant is engaged in occupations of daily living for reinforcement and generalization of new learning.

Evaluation

The participant's score on the Mini-Mental Status Exam was 24 (Folstein, M., et al., 1975). Results of the Unified Parkinson's Disease Rating Scale revealed mild intellectual impairment; periods of sadness; loss of initiative and disinterest in occupations; mildly affected speech; increased salivation; choking on rare occasions; illegible handwriting; slow and clumsy use of utensils for eating; dependence in dressing in areas of placing arms in sleeves and buttoning; increased time required for hygiene; slow and clumsy bed mobility; falling on rare occasions; mild deviations in gait; slight transient tremor; monotone speech; flat affect; slight tremor in right hand; slight rigidity in movements of neck, mild-to-moderate in right upper and lower extremities, and slight in left upper and lower extremities; severely impaired ability to tap thumb with index finger in rapid succession on right and moderately impaired on left; severely impaired ability to open and close both hands in rapid succession and pronation and supination of both forearms; severely decreased endurance in right leg and moderately decreased in left leg; increased time and multiple attempts to complete sit-to-stand transfers; flexed and asymmetric posture; retropulsion with independent recovery; a slow, shuffling gait pattern; and, slow, hesitant, and small amplitude movements (Movement Disorder Society Task Force on Rating Scales for Parkinson's Disease, 2003).

At the onset of the study, the participant's grip strength on the right was 67 pounds and grip strength on the left was 75 pounds. Distance visual acuity using the Snellen Eye Chart revealed a distance visual acuity score of 20/50 and near visual acuity using the Jaeger Eye Test was J.7, which is equivalent to 20/47 using the Snellen Eye Chart. The participant was able to hold a side-by-side, semi-tandem, and tandem stand for 10 seconds respectively. His score on his length of walk test course was 3 meters. The time it took the participant to complete his first usual walk was 62 seconds and his second usual walk was 59 seconds. The participant's fastest 3 meter walk was 4.66 to 6.52 seconds. The participant was able to safely stand up from a chair without the use of his arms. He was able to repeat chair-to-stand transfers 5 times in 23 seconds.

Prior to the onset of the intervention, the participant completed the PDQ-39 Questionnaire (Jenkinson, et al., 2003). He reported occasional difficulty engaging in leisure occupations; often experiences problem with walking 100 yards; occasional problems with mobility within the home; sometimes has difficulty with community mobility; occasionally requires someone to escort him in the community; occasionally worries about falling in public; occasionally feels confined to his home; occasionally experiences difficulty with dressing himself; occasionally has difficulty with handwriting; occasionally has difficulty with cutting his food; occasionally has difficulty with holding a drink in a cup; occasionally feels depressed, tearful, angry, and anxious; occasionally feels the need to hide his symptoms related to

Parkinson's from others; occasionally feels embarrassed in public due to his symptoms associated with Parkinson's; occasionally worries about other's reactions to him; occasionally has problems with close personal relationships; occasionally lacks support from his spouse, family, and/or friends in the ways that he feels he needs; sometimes falls asleep unexpectedly during the day; sometimes has difficulty concentrating when watching television or reading; occasionally feels his memory is poor; occasionally experiences difficulty with his speech and feels unable to communicate with others; occasionally feels ignored by others; experiences occasional muscles spasms; has occasional pain in his joints; and, feels unpleasantly hot or cold. The participant reported slight interest in learning new things; a slight interest in things; a slight concern about his condition; a slight exertion of effort when engaged in occupations; slight need for something to do to occupy his time; no plans or goals for his future; slight motivation; slight amount of energy for occupations of daily living; and, a slight need for "a push to get started."

On The University of Illinois at Chicago Fear of Falling Measure (Velozo & Peterson, 2001), the participant reported feeling very worried about falling when picking up something from the floor and moderately worried about carrying a plate of food, car transfers, walking, using an escalator, climbing stairs, stepping off of a curb, tub transfers, climbing the steps on a bus, standing on a moving bus, using a step stool to reach items in a cupboard, carrying packages up steps, and walking on ice.

The participant completed the Depression Questionnaire (Beck, 1998) prior to the onset of the intervention and reported that he does not find any pleasure in the things that he used to enjoy; that he has lost confidence in himself; that he is less interested in people and things than before; that he has difficulty with making decisions; that he feels worthless compared to others; that he does not have enough energy to do much; that he sleeps more than usual; that he is more irritable than usual; that his appetite is somewhat less than usual, that he cannot concentrate as well as usual; that he is too tired to do a lot of the things that he used to do; and, that he is less interested in sex than he used to be.

The participant's occupational configuration consisted of preparing cereal and fruit for breakfast, reading the newspaper, watching the history channel on television, preparing soup for lunch, taking a nap, making supper, loading the dishwasher, watching the evening news, taking a shower, watching television, and going to bed. During the summer months, the participant reported engaging in yard work.

The participant completed The Washington University Activity Card Sort, Form B (Baum & Edwards, 2001). with patient reporting that he has given up car maintenance; paying the bills; engaging in hand crafts that included woodworking; playing table games; collecting; reading magazines and books; going to the museum and theater; watching movies; bowling; walking; exercising; boating; fishing; traveling; having and attending to parties and picnics and family gatherings; visiting family and friends; and, going to children's activities.

Goal Setting

The participant identified the weekly goals throughout his involvement in the study using the Self Identified Goal Assessment (Melville & Nelson, 2001). The weekly goals identified by the participant using the Self-Identified Goal Assessment included independence in bed mobility; bed, tub, toilet, chair, car, lawnmower and airplane transfers; self care occupations that included buttoning and unbuttoning and donning and doffing shirts and pants, overcoat, and wrist watch; household chores; lawn care; opening and closing containers; reading and comprehending instructions on containers; answering questions; cleaning the garage; working on his car; driving; kneeling and standing during the church service; and, singing at hymns at church.

Occupational Therapy-Based Interventions

The participant successfully completed the six visits of home-based occupational therapy interventions prescribed in the protocol of this study. The evaluation and interventions took place within the context of the naturalistic environment consisting of home and community. The final occupational therapy intervention included the participant's spouse, as both the participant and the occupational therapist agreed that it would be beneficial to review the findings and recommendations that resulted from the participant's involvement in the study with his spouse.

Throughout the interventions, the participant and the occupational therapist completed a variety of occupations that were identified as being meaningful to the participant both in his home, as well as in his local community. Evaluations of the home and community settings were an important component of the intervention.

A sensorimotor approach was utilized as the theoretical framework for this case study. This specialized approach was selected because of the emphasis on the principles related to the use sensory input to facilitate motor output through the proprioceptive, tactile, vestibular, auditory, and visual sensory systems to improve neuroplasticity and decrease falls. This approach suggests that facilitation of the sensory systems to improve motor output be immediately followed by or integrated into occupation for there be an adaptive response and resultant improvement in function.

As the participant in this case study progressed, occupations performed during the intervention became progressively more difficult to include occupations that required multiple steps and/or divided attention in the home and community. The participant was successful in transferring his newly learned approach to the movement to occupations of daily living. A hierarchical approach based on a sensorimotor approach was utilized to guide the intervention, beginning with the basic occupation of "getting out of bed" to the complex occupation of "driving to church."

At the onset of the intervention, the participant was asked to record falls using a daily calendar. Throughout the five intervention sessions, the participant and the occupational therapist performed the routine occupations of daily living that were identified by the participant when administering the occupational configuration. Adaptive devices and durable medical equipment were recommended.

Throughout the six interventions, the participant was instructed in a home program of preparatory occupations that consisted of bilateral overhead reaching; unilateral and bilateral diagonal movements; rotation of upper trunk on lower trunk, lower trunk on upper trunk, and bilateral arm swing; scapular retraction; upper thoracic extension; deep breathing techniques; sit-to-stand transfers; multidirectional sustained movements that included floor-to-ceiling, side-to-side, stepping-and-reaching forwards/sideways/backwards, rocking-and-reach reaching forwards and backwards, rocking and twisting and reaching side-to-side, and functional repetitive movements that included sit-to-stand. This home program was completed at the onset of each intervention as preparatory and purposeful, with the goal of improving posture and alignment and mobility required for safe and efficient performance while engaged in occupations of daily living and independent occupations of daily living. The participant was instructed on strategies for learning to self-monitor his respiration, vocalization and phonation to improve speech intelligibility.

Preparatory and purposeful occupations also included strategies for self-monitoring oral motor control and swallowing, and facial expression. Data indicates that by simultaneously targeting speech and gross motor movements can is complementary to both.

Specific occupations that were performed during intervention included bed mobility; sit-to-stand and stand-pivot transfers; tub transfers; toilet transfers; chair transfers, including reclining rocker in the living room, where participant most likes to sit; upper and lower body dressing, including suitcoat and overcoat and suit and tie for church; reaching for items in kitchen cupboards and shelves in refrigerator; simple meal preparation for lunch; carrying garbage out to the road; sweeping the garage floor; reaching for tools on garage shelves; opening and closing hood of automobile; car transfers; lawnmower transfers; cutting the grass using a riding lawnmower; fastening his seatbelt in his car; backing his car out of the garage and down his driveway; driving car to church; parking at church; accessing church; kneeling in church pew; ascending and descending the steps to the altar at church; kneeling at altar for communion; and, practicing singing familiar church hymns while at church.

Together, the participant and therapist collaborated to make some changes to his home. The adaptive equipment recommended included reachers, a leg lift, and a button hook. The durable medical equipment that was recommended included a tub seat, hand-held shower, a raised toilet with safety frame, and a grab bar mounted on the passenger frame of participant's small engine airplane, and, a push broom.

The environmental recommendations included removing all throw rugs from the participant's home, replacing rolling and swiveling kitchen chairs that did not have armrests with chairs that are stationary and that have armrests; replacing his swivel rocking chair with a stable and supportive easy chair; opening sliding door on airplane hangar; a railing on the church alter, a push-button door opener on the door of the church, and a second handicapped parking sign in the church parking lot so that each space would have a sign. Specific strategies included keeping knot in tie to avoid having to tie it each time he dresses for church; swinging overcoat over his opposite shoulder when donning; turning car around in drive prior versus backing car down driveway; sit versus stand to sort tools.

At the end of the sixth intervention session, the occupational therapist provided the participant and his spouse with a written summary of the recommendations that had been made throughout the course of the six weeks.

Included in the recommendations, was that the participant complete an occupational therapy evaluation to assess his safety for driving.

Evidence-Based Outcomes

The occupational therapist called the participant two weeks, six weeks, and six months after the last visit to assess the effectiveness of the recommendations and to answer any questions that the participant had. During these calls, the occupational therapist and the participant worked together to modify the recommendations as needed.

Upon completion of the six week intervention, the participant reported independence in bed mobility; independence in bed mobility using a leg lift, bed transfers, tub transfers using a tub seat and grab bar, toilet transfers with use of a raised toilet seat with safety frame, chair transfers from stable easy chair, car transfers, lawnmower transfers, and airplane transfers with grab bar mounted on the frame of the door; independence in occupations that included: donning and doffing shirts using a button hook; donning and doffing pants using button hook and reachers; donning his overcoat and suit coat; donning and doffing his wrist watch; household chores; lawn care using his riding lawnmower; opening and closing containers during meal preparation; reading and comprehending instructions on containers; answering questions; cleaning the garage using a push broom; working on his car; modified driving only to church on Sundays; kneeling and standing during the church service; singing hymns at church; accessing door to church; and, ascending and descending the altar steps in order to receive communion at church.

References

Baum, M., & Edwards, D. (2001). *Activity Card Sort*. St. Louis, MO: Washington University School of Medicine.

Beck, A.T., Steer, R.A., & Brown, G.K. (1996). *Beck Depression Inventory: Second edition*. The Psychological Corporation: San Antonio, TX. .

Folstein, M. F., Folstein, S. E., & McHugh, P. F. (1975). Mini mental state: A practical method for grading the cognitive state of patients for the clinician. *Journal of Psychiatric Research, 12*, 189-198.

Melville, L. L., & Nelson, D. L. (1996, 2001). Melville-Nelson Self-Identified Goals Assessment. Retrieved at http://www.utoledo.edu/hshs/ot/melville.html

Movement Disorder Society Task Force on Rating Scales for Parkinson's Disease (2003). The Unified Parkinson's Disease Rating Scale (UPDRS): Status and recommendations. *Movement Disorders*, *18*, 738-750.

Velozo, C. A., & Peterson, E. W. (2001). Developing meaningful fear of falling measures for community dwelling elderly. *American Journal of Physical Medicine & Rehabilitation, 80*, 662-673.

In: Accidental Falls
Editor: Brenda Evans

ISBN: 978-1-63483-228-1

Chapter 4

SELF-PERCEIVED HEALTH AND THE RISK OF FALLING IN A BRAZILIAN COMMUNITY SAMPLE

Patricia Morsch[*]
Institute of Geriatrics and Gerontology,
Pontifical Catholic University of Rio Grande do Sul, Porto Alegre, Brazil

ABSTRACT

In Brazil and in the United States, the prevalence of falls is approximately 30%. A lot of measures have been adopted trying to reduce this rate; however, the number of older adults who fall is still rising. Falling is associated with increased disability rates, as well as hospital and nursing home admissions. Research has identified many risk factors for falling, including physical and environmental hazards. In addition, as many chronic diseases older adults present, higher is the risk of falling. Self-perceived health has been used in research as a good indicator of individuals' actual health. Using a secondary dataset the relationship between self-perceived health and falls was tested in community dwelling older adults from the state of Rio Grande do Sul, Brazil. The data were used to test whether self-perceived health is associated with falling, controlling for sociodemographic variables (age, gender and monthly household income). Analysis was conducted using bivariate cross tabulation and noting of chi-square values. To sum up,

[*] Email: patriciamorsch@hotmail.com

self-perceived health has a relationship with falls and this is an important finding since inquiring self-perceived health is a simple and fast measure that might be useful in identifying older adults at risk of falling.

INTRODUCTION

Older adults are the fastest growing age group worldwide (Coimbra, Ricci, Coimbra & Costallat, 2010). In Brazil, according to data from 2010 Census report, the proportion of older adults (65 and older) increased from 4.8% in 1991 to 5.9% in 2000 and 7.4% in 2010 (IBGE, 2011). Approximately 16% of the Brazilian population over 60 years old live in the state of Rio Grande do Sul. This state has one of the highest percentages of older adults in Brazil (IBGE, 2011; IBGE, 2009).

With the increase of this population, a wide range of problems affecting older adults deserve special attention, including falls. Even though there is little agreement, on the best definition of falls, one of the most used in the literature is: "unintentionally coming to the ground or some lower level and other than as a consequence of sustaining a violent blow, loss of consciousness, sudden onset of paralysis as in stroke or an epileptic seizure" (Kellogg International Working Group on the Prevention of Falls, 1987 as cited in Lord et al, 2007, p.3).

The high incidence of falls among older adults highlights the importance of this topic; in Brazil and in the United States, approximately 30% of the older adult population falls each year and this percentage increases to 50% for the oldest old (Coimbra et al., 2010; Tinnetti et al., 1988). Falling can lead to severe consequences for the elderly as they are an important cause of health problems and psychological impairment.

Not only older adults suffer the negative consequences of a fall, it also affects older adults' families as falling can cause immobility, dependence (Pereira, Vogelaere & Baptista, 2008), a fear of falling, institutionalization, and increased mortality risk (Brasil, 2010; Roe et al, 2009). Falls accounts for 4% of hospital admissions, 40% of death related to injury and 1% of total death in older adults (Lord, Sherrington, Menz & Klosem, 2007).

Falling also affect health care systems. In the United States, costs related to falls were $ 20.2 billion in 1994 and are predicted to increase to $ 32.4 billion by 2020. The Brazilian health care system spends almost R$ 51 million annually to treat fractures in older adults who fell. Fractures and hospital admission due to falls in older adults has increased; research suggests that 20%

of older adults have some kind of injury, needing special care, after experiencing a fall (Coimbra et al., 2010; Brasil, 2012). Therefore, falls lead to great demands on health care systems (Stel, Smit, Pluijm & Lips, 2004).

Falls are often described as accidents; however, there are many causes related to them and, consequently, these events cannot be considered a random occurrence (Lord et al., 2007). Usually, a single fall is caused by environmental hazards. However, when older adults experience multiple falls, it is usually due to underlying chronic conditions (Lach, 2005). More than 60% of all falls experienced by elders are caused by interaction of multiple factors (Rose, 2008). The risk of falling and fractures are related to the number of chronic conditions presented by older adults; risk becomes higher when more risk factors interact. In addition, research suggests that falls are more common among individuals who present physical frailty, reduced emotional support and perceptions of poor health (Sharaf & Ibrahim, 2008). Self-perceived health has been used as a good indicator of actual health status and functional ability in older adults (Borges et al, 2014).

Overall, institutionalized older adults and those with diseases affecting muscle strength, balance and gait are more likely to fall, as well as women in the post-menopausal period (Brasil, 2012; Coimbra et al., 2010). Additionally, the risk of falling increases remarkably after the age of 65, and continues to increase steadily with age (Coimbra et al., 2010).

Risk factors of falls can be divided into two main categories: intrinsic and extrinsic (Walker, Porock & Timmons, 2011). Intrinsic factors are physiological factors, including visual and hearing impairment, depression, cardiovascular and neurological diseases and musculoskeletal problems. Extrinsic factors are related to the environment and include uneven pathways, slippery floor surfaces, bad lighting, loose rugs, telephone wires and stairways without handrails. Medication intake is also an important extrinsic risk factor for falls (Walker, Porock & Timmons, 2011; Pereira, Vogelaere & Baptista, 2010; Keller 2009). Roe et al. (2009) suggest that alcohol consumption is an important extrinsic risk factor which has to be better addressed in the older adult population. Some authors classify behavior as a third category in the risk factors for falls, including emotions and actions in the daily life in this group (Fabrício, Rodrigues & Costa Júnior, 2004; Messias & Neves, 2009).

Approximately 30% to 40% of falls are preventable and the most effective way to do so is by identifying individuals with risk factors and having them participate in prevention activities (Sjosten, Vaapio & Kivela, 2008). There are many methods and programs to prevent falls available, such as exercise programs and assessment of older adults' environment. However, there is little agreement about which of the approaches work best. Some authors believe that the focus of prevention should be on changing health behavior and modifiable risk factors (Walker, Porock & Timmons, 2011). However, others suggest that a multidisciplinary approach is very important for fall prevention, since falls usually have multiple causes (Pereira, Vogealere & Baptista, 2008). Dickinson et al. (2011) state that for any program, older adults have to commit, attend, and participate in the activities to achieve its benefits. These researchers found different barriers and facilitators to participation in fall prevention program. Understanding what older adults' motivations and expectations are seems to be crucial for fall prevention programs success (Dickinson et al., 2011).

Even with the wide range of fall prevention programs and knowledge related to falls, the prevalence of falls has not diminished. This chapter aims to verify the relationship between falling and self-perceived health, as it can be a useful questioning to screen older adults at risk for falling.

Methods

This chapter focused on community dwelling older men and women, over the age of 60 years old, living in the state of Rio Grande do Sul, Brazil. It was conducted secondary analysis of a dataset that was collected by a private company for the Pontifical Catholic University at Porto Alegre and the Public Health School with a state grant. The sample consists of community dwelling older adults aged 60 years old and older, living in urban and rural areas of the state of the Rio Grande do Sul. From the 497 cities in the state of Rio Grande do Sul, 39 were randomly selected to be part of the study. This was done with a multi-pronged sampling strategy that involved multi-cluster sampling, systematic sampling of households within the cluster of the neighborhood, and a random selection of an older individual within the household. In each city, census sectors were identified using the National Census information and randomly selected as well. The main project was entitled "The profile of older adults from the Rio Grande do Sul state," which methods were fully described previously elsewhere (Pereira et al, 2013; Morsch et al, 2015).

For the purposes of this chapter, only demographic questions as well as self-perceived health and fall history was used. The dependent variable, history of falls, is identified with a question which asks if the respondent has experienced a fall in the last 12 months. If the answer was yes, it was asked how many times approximately. This variable was recoded separating individuals that did not fall in the last year from the ones who did fall.

Individuals were included in the missing category if they answered they did not know if they fell or not.

The independent variables are demographic information, age (divided in age groups of 10 years old), gender, race (white, black and other), monthly household income [based on the Brazilian minimum wage, which was R$ 510 (US$296.77) in 2011]. Categories for this variable are no income, low income (0.1–2 minimum wages), medium income (2.1–4 minimum wages) and high income (more than or equal to 4.1 minimum wages).

The last independent variable related to the demographic factors is educational attainment (illiterate - no education; low education – knowledge but no school to complete elementary school; medium/high education: above elementary school). Self-perceived health was identified by a multiple-choice question which asked respondents to rate their own health as very good, good, average, poor or very poor. If a proxy responded to this question, the interviewer was instructed to mark "not applicable." In the health group, the variable self-perceived health remained the same regarding the categories named very good, good and average. The last category was recoded into poor and it comprises self-perceived health status reported as poor and very poor.

The bivariate relationship between self-perceived health and falls was tested by using a cross tabulation table and noting the chi square statistic. Results were controlled for gender, income and age by including these demographic variables in the bivariate model. Because the analysis is based on cross-sectional data it is only possible to look at whether there was a relationship between self-perceived health and falls; it was not possible to infer causal relationship. For the analysis, the IBM SPSS Statistics 19.0 package was used.

Results

In order to describe the sample of the present chapter, frequencies are described in Table 1. It consisted of 6968 older adults, including 3617 women (51.9%) and 3351 (48.1%) men. Approximately half of the older adults in the sample are in the age group of 60-69 years old (51.9%), more than half are white (69.2%) and most of the respondents have low income (48.8%) and low educational attainment (46.8%) and just 9.2% of the sample had a fall in the last year. Even though research suggests that 30% of older adults fall in Brazil each year, 9.2% is still a considerable number. It can be suggested that most of the individuals from the study sample have generally good health status. More than half of the respondents reported their self-perceived health as good (60.7%).

Table 1. Frequencies of all studied variables

Variables	Frequencies	%
Age		
60-69	3616	51.9%
70-79	2416	34.7%
80 +	929	13.3%
Missing	7	0.1%
Gender		
Female	3617	51.9%
Male	3351	48.1%
Race		
White	4822	69.2%
Black	1793	25.7%
Other	39	0.6%
Missing	314	4.5%
Education Attainment		
Illiterate	655	9.4%
Low	3261	46.8%
Medium	2017	28.9%
High	802	11.5%
Household Income		
Low	3403	48.8%
Medium	2071	20.7%
High	781	11.2%
Missing	713	10.2%
Falls		
No	6180	88.7%
Yes	640	9.2%
Missing	148	2.1%
Self-perceived health		
Very Good	613	8.8%
Good	4228	60.7%
Average	1705	24.5%
Poor	342	4.9%
Missing	80	1.1%

Source: "The profile of older adults from the Rio Grande do Sul state," 2011.

Table 2 shows the relationship between the demographic data studied (i.e., age, gender, race, educational attainment and household income), self-perceived health and falls. It shows that apart from race, all the other variables have a significant relationship with falling. Considering self-perceived health, it is important to point out that individuals who perceived themselves as having poor health were more likely to have fallen than ones who perceived their health as good.

Table 2. Relationship between demographic data, self-perceived health and falling

Variable	Had Fallen	%	Crosstabs Total	χ^2	p value
Age			n = 6813	143.40	***
60-69	213	5.9%			
70-79	265	11.3%			
80 +	162	18.4%			
Gender			n = 6820	14.72	***
Female	378	10.7%			
Male	262	8%			
Race			n = 6526	0.87	n.s.
White	457	9.6%			
Black	160	9.1%			
Other	5	12.8%			
Education Attainment			n = 6595	28.18	***
Table 6 (continued)					
Illiterate	86	13.4%			
Low	334	10.5%			
Medium	143	7.2%			
High	67	8.4%			
Household Income			n = 6125	6.18	*
Low	343	10.2%			
Medium	164	8.2%			
High	72	9.4%			
Self-perceived health			n = 6745	270.60	***
Very Good	27	4.4%			
Good	241	5.8%			
Average	276	17%			
Poor	75	23%			

Source: "The profile of older adults from the Rio Grande do Sul state," 2011

* $p < .05$

*** $p < .001$

n.s. = not significant.

In order to further investigate the relationship between falls and self-perceived health, results were controlled for age, gender and income (Table 3). None of the additional variables affected the results. It can be suggested that self-perceived health have a significant relationship with falling across categories of age, gender and income.

Table 3. Relationship between falls and self-perceived health controlling for age, gender and income

	Self-Perceived Health χ^2	Significance
Age		
60-69	95.34	***
70-79	100.64	***
80+	30.02	***
Gender		
Male	76.92	***
Female	214.35	***
Household Income		
Low	112.75	***
Medium	84.47	***
High	40.61	***

Source: "The profile of older adults from the Rio Grande do Sul state," 2011.
*** $p < .001$.

Research about falling in older adults is broad, and a lot is already known especially about physical conditions and environmental factors that predispose for falls among older adults. Even with the large amount of studies, the number of older adults experiencing a fall is still rising. Therefore, it is important to find simple ways to identify older adults at higher risk of falling.

Self-perceived health has been associated with actual health status and compliance with positive health behaviors, including participation in physical activities (Dogra, 2011). As the relationship between self-perceived health and falls was strong in this chapter, it may be suggested that, a good way to screen older adults' risk for falling and also adherence to fall prevention programs is by asking their self-perceived health.

According to Davis et al. (2007) the ability to keep good thoughts and a positive outlook on life may promote optimal functioning and high quality of life in adults. In addition, Levy, Slade and Kasl (2002) found that, not only self-perceived health, but also self-perception of aging predicts functional health over time. These researchers suggest that older adults who have a positive outlook about aging report better functional health than those with a negative perception, after controlling for baseline measures of functional health, self-rated health, age, gender, loneliness, race and socioeconomic status. It has been also suggested that self-perception of aging has a greater impact in survival and longevity for older adults than gender, socio economic status, loneliness, and functional health (Levy, Slade, Kasl & Kunkel, 2002). These outcomes highlight the importance of considering self-perceved health and aging and its impact in older adults' health, well-being and the relationship with falling.

In addition, a low sense of control over their own lives can lead older adults to have low motivation for action, which might be related to lack of compliance in good health behaviors and therefore, impact health negatively (Cotter & Lachman, 2010). Positive emotions are also related to increased cognitive resources, including improved feelings of self-efficacy and increased understanding and willingness to avoid risky behaviors. In addition, a positive outlook is associated with improved ability to maintain social relations and positive health behaviors (Davis et al., 2007). These findings suggest that if older adults adhere to good health behaviors, they might improve their self-perceived health and, ultimately, reduce the risk of falls.

Apart from the relevant findings it is very important to point out the reduced number of older adults who reported falling in this chapter. As previously stated, 30% of older adults fall each year, and just 9.2% of the current sample reported falling. Perhaps the lack of definition of a fall may have played a role in the way older adults interpreted and answered the question. In addition, the way the question was worded, asking if the individual "fell to the ground" may have caused different interpretations as well. The possibility of answering "do not know" may have discouraged older adults to think about it and encouraged them to give a simple and faster answer. Also, the majority of respondents in this sample were in the young-old group (60 through 69 years old). Talbot et al. (2005) found that 21% of older adults from 46 through 65 years old fell in the two years of their study. As suggested by these authors and these findings, the likelihood of falling increases with age. In addition, Ruthig et al. (2007) suggest that younger older adults might experience less serious falls or recover more rapidly from their effects when compared to the oldest old group. Therefore, younger older adults may be at risk of under-reporting falls.

Another suggestion for the lower frequency of falls in this population is that falling is usually a very sensitive topic for older adults to talk about and they might deny having experienced a fall. Research has found that in older ages, falls can represent loss of control of their own body and many older adults relate falling to a loss of dignity (Mahler & Sarvimaki, 2010). In their qualitative study regarding falling and its meaning for older men and women,

Mahler and Sarvimaki (2010) found that participants avoided talking about falls and one participant, at the beginning of the interview, totally denied having experienced a fall, even though participants were selected from fall-registration sheets and from a course in fall prevention.

Self-perceived health is a self-reported measure, which can be a potential limitation for this chapter results. For individuals with some kind of cognitive impairment, a proxy was designated to respond to the questionnaire, which could have been a limitation of the data collected. However, after careful consideration of the dataset, the small number of proxies used (1.3%) did not influence the findings. Another limitation of the study is that a causal relationship between self-perceived health and falls cannot be inferred because of lack of temporal data.

Further research should be developed to verify a causal relationship between falls and self-perceived health. Conducting longitudinal studies where it is possible to untangle the order of occurrence of events would be very important, so that it is possible to discriminate cause and effect and target them specifically in fall prevention programs. Also, it would be interesting to analyze the relationship between these variables in different groups, living in different areas of Brazil or different countries, since older adults may face different psychological or social factors in different areas. The Rio Grande do Sul state, is in the southern area of Brazil, it was colonized by Europeans and have one of the best quality of life status in the country. It is probably very different from the states in the North of Brazil, for example.

To summarize, falls are an important problem among the older adult population and fall prevention programs are crucial to reduce the burden a fall can cause for older individuals, their families, and the public system. Identifying factors that are associated with falling can improve the efficiency of fall prevention programs. From the results of this study, self-perceived health has a significant relationship with falls. Therefore, asking older adults' self-perceived health might be a good tool to screen older adults at risk of falling and having them to engage in fall prevention programs.

References

Brasil. Portal Brasil. Quedas. 2012. Retrieved from: http://www.brasil.gov.br /saude/2012/04/quedas.

Borges, A.M., Santos, G., Kummer, J.A., Fior, L., Dal Molin, V., Wibelinger, L.M. (2014). Autopercepção de saúde em idosos residentes em um município do interior do Rio Grande do Sul. *Revista Brasileira de Geriatria e Gerontologia, 17*(1), 79-86.

Coimbra, A.M., Ricci, N.A., Coimbra, I.B. & Costallat, L.T. (2010). Falls in the elderly of the Family Health Program. *Archives of Gerontology and Geriatrics, 51*, 317 – 322.

Cotter, K.A. & Lachman, M.E. (2010). Psychosocial and behavioral contributors to health: Age-related increases in physical disability are reduced by physical fitness. *Psychology and Health, 25* (7), 805 – 820.

Davis, M.C., Zautra, A.J., Johnson, L.M., Murray, K.E, & Okvat, H.A. (2007). Psychosocial stress, emotion regulation, and resilience among older adults. In C. Aldwin, C. Park & A. Spiro III (Ed) *Handbook of health psychology and aging,* (pp. 250–266). New York, NY: The Guilford Press.

Dickinson, A., Machen, I., Horton, K., Jain, D., Maddex, T. & Cove, J. (2011). Fall prevention in the community: what older people say they need. *British Journal of Community Nursing, 16* (4), 174 – 180.

Dogra, S. (2011). Better self-perceived health is associated with lower odds of physical inactivity in older adults with chronic diseases. *Human Kinetics, 19,* 322 – 335.

Fabrício, S.C.C, Rodrigues, R.A.P. & Costa Júnior, M.L. Falls among older adults seen at a São Paulo State public hospital: causes and consequences. (2004). *Rev Saúde Públ, 38* (1), 93 – 99.

IBGE (2009). Population and Households – PNAD 2009 - Summary of Indicators. Retrieved from: http://www.ibge.gov.br/estadosat/temas.php?sigla=rs&tema=pnad_2013

IBGE (2011). 2010 Census first final results: Brazil has a population of 190.755.799 residents. Retrieved from: http://censo2010.ibge.gov.br/noticias-censo?%20view=noticia&id=1&idnoticia=%201866&t=primeiros-resultados-definitivos-censo-2010-populacao-brasil-190-755-799-pessoas

Keller, J.M. (2009). A holistic approach to developing fall-prevention programs for community dwelling older adults. *Activities, adaptation & aging, 33*, 223 – 239.

Lach, H.W. (2005). Incidence and Risk Factors for Developing Fear of Falling in Older Adults. *Public Health Nursing, 22* (1), 45-52.

Levy, B.R., Slade, M.D. & Kasl, S.V. (2002). Longitudinal benefit of positive self-perceptions of aging on functional health. *Journals of Gerontology: Psychological Sciences, 57b* (5), 409 - 417.

Levy, B.R., Slade, M.D., Kasl, S.V. & Kunkel, S.R. (2002). Longevity increased by positive self-perceptions of aging. *Journals of Personality and Social Psychology, 83* (2), 261 - 270.

Lord, S., Sherrington, C., Menz, H. & Close, J. (2007). *Falls* in Older People: Risks factors and strategies for prevention. New York: *Cambridge University Press*.

Mahler, M. & Sarvimaki, A. (2010). Indispensable chairs and comforting cushions – Falls and the meaning of falls in six older persons lives. *Journal of Aging Studies, 24,* 88 – 95.

Messias, M.G.& Neves, R.F. A influência de fatores comportamentais e ambientais domésticos nas quedas em idosos. (2009). *Rev Bras Geriatr Gerontol, 12* (2), 275-282.

Morsch, P., Shenk, D., Bós, A.J.G. The relationship between falls and psychological well-being in a Brazilian community sample. (2015). *J. Cross Cult. Gerontol, 30* (1), 119-127.

Pereira, C.L., Vogelaere, P. & Baptista, F. (2008). Role of physical activity in the prevention of falls and their consequences in the elderly. *Eur. Rev. Aging. Phys. Act, 5*, 51 – 58.

Pereira, G.N., Morsch, P.M, Lopes, D.C.G., Trevisan, M.D., Ribeiro A....Bós, A.J.G. (2013). Fatores socioambientais associados à ocorrência de quedas em idosos, *Ciênc. Saúde Colet, 18* (12), 3507-3514.

Roe, B., Howell, F., Riniotis, K., Beech, R., Crome, P. & Ong, B.N. (2009). Older people and falls: health status, quality of life, lifestyle, care networks, prevention and views on service use following a recent fall. *Journal of Clinical Nursing, 18*, 2261 – 2272.

Rose, D. (2008). Preventing falls among older adults: No "one size suits all" intervention strategy. *Journal of Rehabilitation Research & Development, 45* (8), 1153–1166.

Ruthig, J.C., Chipperfield J.G., Newall N.E, Perry R.P. & Hall, N.C. (2007). Detrimental effects of falling on health and well-being in later life: The mediating roles of perceived control and optimism. *Journal of Health Psychology, 12* (2), 231 – 248.

Sharaf, A. & Ibrahim, H. (2008). Physical and psychosocial correlates of fear of falling among older adults in assisted living facilities. *Journal of Gerontological Nursing, 34* (12), 27-35.

Sjosten, N., Vaapio, S. & Kivela, S.-L. (2008). The effects of fall prevention trials on depressive symptoms and fear of falling among the aged: A systematic review. *Aging & Mental Health, 12* (1), 30-46.

Stel, V.S., Smit, J.H., Pluijm, S.M. & Lips, P. (2004). Consequences of falling in older men and women and risk factors for health service use and functional decline. *Age and Ageing, 33* (1), 58-65.

Walker, W., Porock, D. & Timmons, S. (2011). The importance of identity in falls prevention. *Nursing Older People, 23* (2), 21 – 26.

Talbot, L.A., Musiol R.J., Witham E.K. & Metter E.J. (2005). Falls in young, middle-aged and older community dwelling adults: perceived caused, environmental factos and injury. *BMC Public Health, 5* (86).

Tinetti, M.E., Speechley, M. & Ginter, S.F. (1988). Risk factors for falls among elderly persons living in the community. *The New England Journal of Medicine, 319* (26), 1701 – 1707.

In: Accidental Falls
Editor: Brenda Evans

ISBN: 978-1-63483-228-1

Chapter 5

PRACTICAL DESIGN SEARCH FOR OPTIMAL FLOOR SURFACE FINISHES TO PREVENT FALL INCIDENTS

In-Ju Kim

Department of Industrial Engineering, College of Engineering
King Saud University, Riyadh, Saudi Arabia

ABSTRACT

Increasing traction properties of the floor surface would be desirable as a general rule, but a very high level of slip-resistance may impede safe and comfortable ambulation. There is lack of evidences whether traction properties are linearly correlated with surface features of the floor or what levels of floor surface finishes are required to effective control of slipperiness. It is also scarce to find studies and/or guidelines on the operational ranges of floor surface roughness required for optimal slip-resistance performance. The objectives of this chapter are to investigate the effects of floor surface finishes on slip-resistance performance under different environmental and shoe-type conditions, and identify operational ranges of floor surface roughness as practical design information for the prevention of fall incidents. A theory model of three operative zones was suggested to characterize functional levels of floor surface roughness on slip-resistance performance. To test the theory model, dynamic friction tests were conducted using 3 shoes and 9 floor specimens under 2 lubricated environments: wet and soapy conditions. The test results showed that significant effects of floor-type on dynamic friction coefficient (DFC) were found in both lubricated conditions. As compared to the floor-type effects, shoe-type effects were relatively small. Slip-resistance performance was significantly affected by and well correlated with the floor surface roughness under the soapy environment. Polynomial regression analyses amongst the floor surface roughness, DFCs and environments allowed to estimating operational ranges for optimal slip-resistance performance. Under the soapy environment, floor surfaces with 17 and 52 μm in *Ra* roughness parameter most likely represented the lower and upper bounds of the operational ranges. The test result also identified that the soapsuds-covered soapy floors required rougher surface finishes than the wet ones in their lower boundary roughness range. However, there were lack of correlations between the surface roughness and slip-resistance properties under the wet surface condition. The current study suggests that designs for the floor surface finishes would require different levels of surface roughness for different types of environmental conditions to effectively control slippery walking environments.

Keywords: Design of operational levels, floor surfaces, slip-resistance, slips and falls, wet and soapy conditions

INTRODUCTION

Sip and fall incidents are the second leading personal injury and have been recognized as a major threat to the safety of individuals not only in industry but also in daily living (Yeoh et al., 2013). Slip and fall incidents are vulnerable to the elderly people and are one of the major health risks that affect their quality of life and independent living. Falls and fall-related injuries are amongst the most serious and common medical problems experienced by the older population with approximately 28% of community-dwelling older adults experiencing at least one fall a year (Kelsey et al., 2012). Importance of the issue has been recognized due to the magnitude of problems and associated costs. There have been prolonged efforts to understand the main causes of such incidents in order to reduce their frequencies and severities.

Although many elements are involved in the slip and fall incidents, footpaths and walkways seem to have a major effect on safe ambulation of the pedestrians. Pedestrian surfaces should be constructed to provide comfortable walking environments and good traction performance against any slippery condition. They also should deliver optimal slip-resistance qualities throughout their lifetimes. Whilst supporting and controlling slip-resistance properties of the floor surfaces would be desirable as a general rule, a specific problem arising in the real world' walking environments is that the slip-resistance of floors and floor coverings deteriorates over time owing to material ageing, surface wear, soiling, and maintenance (Leclercq and Saulnier, 2002). Derler et al. (2008) investigated the shift of friction coefficients for various floor coverings and different test sites over a period of 30 months, in order to study the short- and long-term effects of use and maintenance in detail. It was found that mechanical abrasion and coating by care products lead to the continuous reduction of slip-resistance, a typical outcome for many floor surfaces in use. These results were confirmed by field studies in which the friction of floors and floor coverings were investigated at different test sites; mechanical wear, soiling and maintenance strongly affected the slip-resistance, and the complex interplay of these factors could lead to considerable local variations of the surface properties (Chang et al., 2003, Chang et al., 2008 and Li et al., 2004).

The recent literature also has stressed the importance of surface texture on slip-resistance assessments. A number of surface roughness parameters were measured to identify correlations between the surface roughness and slip-resistance properties (Kim & Smith, 2000 & 2003; Chang, 2001 & 2002; Kim et al., 2001; Kim, 2004a & b, 2006a & b; Kim and Nagata, 2008a &b; Kim et al., 2013; Kim, 2015). Those studies reported that surface roughness on the shoes and floors significantly affected slip-resistance performance. Surface roughness offers drainage spaces to avoid squeeze film formations under contaminated environments. For example, tread patterns on the heel surface could improve traction properties by providing void spaces for the removal of lubricants and leading to an increase in direct contact with the floor surface. Therefore, macro-roughness or tread patterns are commonly designed into the shoe heel/sole areas, but they become ineffective quickly after being worn.

However, floor surfaces seem to provide better effects on slip-resistance performance than shoes because floor finishes may offer sharper, taller and tougher asperities in their surface features than shoe ones (Kim et al., 2001; Kim, 2004a & b). Although intensifying slip-resistance properties of the floor surfaces would be desirable as a general rule, a very high level of traction or slip-resistance may impede safe and comfortable ambulation (Chaffin et al., 1992). Moreover, maintaining and/or increasing surface roughness of the floors and floor coverings require high processing costs.

Despite considerable experimental and analytical research on slip and falls incidents, no simple concept and/or theoretical model has been developed to explore the effect of floor surface finishes on slip-resistance performance. It is also hard to find any definitive studies and design information on operational levels of floor surface roughness required for optimal slip-resistance performance. There are no internationally accepted guidelines and design data on operational levels of floor surface finishes for effective controls of slip-resistance functioning. Therefore, it is necessary to develop a method which can provide practical information on floor surface finishes for efficient control of slip-resistance performance under a range of walking environments.

This study aims to investigate the effects of floor surface finishes on slip-resistance properties and identify operational levels of floor surface roughness for optimal slip-resistance performance under a range of slippery environments. To achieve this aim, the present chapter extends previous findings on operational ranges of the floor surface roughness under different walking environments: tap water-covered wet and soapsuds-covered soapy conditions. The main approach was based on the theory model and concept developed by Kim and colleagues (2013). It is expected that collected information on operative ranges of floor surface roughness under diverse walking environments would help to develop practical design information and future guidelines for floor surface finishes required to prevent pedestrian slip and fall incidents.

THEORY DEVELOPMENT

Main Hypothesis

Friction actions are the results of extremely complex interactions between the surface and near-surface regions of two materials in contact. Physical, chemical, and mechanical properties in the surface and near-surface regions may well differ from the corresponding bulk properties of parent materials (Kim and Nagata, 2008b). In addition, these surface and near-surface regions could change radically as a result of interactions of the surface molecules with their environments and with each other throughout the course of repetitive friction processes (Kim and Nagata, 2008b). Hence, it would be necessary to investigate tribo-physical behaviours between the shoe heel and floor surface and their interactions on slip-resistance properties.

Almost all surfaces are rough on the molecular level and variations in the surface profiles could be represented by a random arrangement of peaks and valleys or asperities. When a shoe heel is loaded against a floor, it could be assumed that two surfaces initially touch only at tiny discrete areas where their highest asperities are in contact, as illustrated in Figure 1(a). A local pressure at the contact regions would be high enough to cause plastic deformation of the heel asperities even at the lightest load because an elastic modulus of the shoe heel would be significantly less than that of the floor surface. Hence, its contact mechanism would be an interlocking status as shown in Figure 1(b) with a magnified format. If the shoe heel slides on the floor surface, then the heel surface would be ruptured, deformed and ploughed by the wedge-shaped hard asperities of the floor surface. In this model, peak heights of the floor surface would be a vital factor affecting the heel contact-sliding mechanism. Therefore, high-peak related roughness parameters of the floor surface and their effects on slip-resistance properties are mainly considered in this chapter.

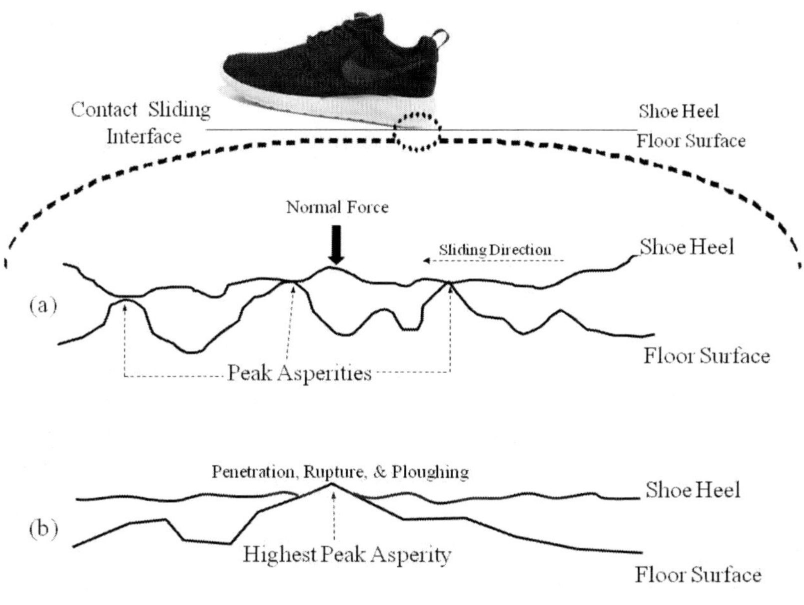

Figure 1.

For the high-peak related roughness parameters, *Rt* (maximum peak-to-valley height) and *Rtm* (maximum mean peak-to-valley height) are considered with *Ra* (centre line average), which is the most widely used roughness parameter (Thomas, 1999; Bewoor & Kulkarni, 2009). These three roughness parameters have been commonly used for assessing the effects of floor surface roughness on slip-resistance performance (Harris and Shaw, 1988; Proctor, 1993; Manning and Jones, 1994; Kim and Smith, 2000, 2003; Chang et al.,

2001; Kim et al., 2001; Leclercq and Saulnier, 2002; Kim, 2004a & b; Li et al., 2004; Kim and Nagata, 2008a & b; Kim et al., 2013; Kim, 2015). Details of the three roughness parameters are found in the literature (BSI, 1988; ISO, 1998; Kim and Smith, 2000; Chang et al., 2001).

Floor Surface Model for Operational Levels

It is hypothesized that floor surface roughness impacts a DFC in a non-linear manner and its effect can be characterized by three operative zones: initial low-growth (Zone 1), mid steady-growth (Zone 2), and top no-growth or peak (Zone 3) as suggested in Figure 2. In the Zone 1, multiple friction mechanisms such as adhesion, abrasion, ploughing, and fatigue are involved and the interlocking is not effective (Kim, 2015). The Zone 2 reflects a dominance of the interlocking mechanism where a linear relationship may be valid whilst the Zone 3 indicates the exhaustion of the interlocking mechanism ("no further benefit").

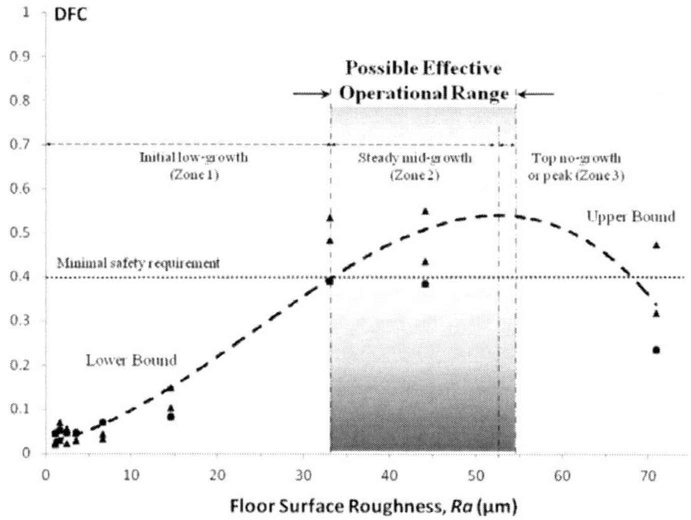

Figure 2.

For practical design purposes, it would be beneficial to find the most effective levels ("operational range") of floor surface roughness, which corresponds to the DFC steady-growth zone. The lower bound of the operational range would be determined by the AS/NZS safety requirement of DFC > 0.4 (AS/NZS 4663, 2004), whilst the upper bound of the operational range would be at surface roughness scales that do not provide further benefit to DFC values (Zone 3).

METHODS

Dynamic Friction Tester

A pendulum-type dynamic friction tester was used to measure slip-resistance properties between a shoe and floor specimen as shown in Figure 3. This test rig consists of two hydraulic systems with an attached artificial foot, a force component transducer (Kistler 3-Component Dynamometer, type 9257A), an angular displacement transducer, and a desktop computer (Kim et al., 2013). This tester simulates movements and loadings of the foot during heel strikes and initial-slips, and quantitatively determines slip-resistance in terms of a dynamic friction coefficient (DFC). The tester's setup values could be adjusted to cover various parameters taken from human walking trials such as a heel contact angle, vertical load, and its rate of increase and sliding speed (Kim et al., 2013). To adjust the heel contact angle, tapered shims were inserted between the base of the pendulum and the last on which the shoe was mounted. The vertical load was set by the length of the pendulum adjusted by two nuts. Some fine adjustment to the vertical load was also possible by a pressure control on the oil fed to the vertical hydraulic cylinder. The sliding speed was set by a flow control valve. In this tester, the test shoe was firmly attached to the last and mounted at the end of the pendulum mechanism. In order to minimize any movement, the shoe specimen was nailed to the last.

The floor specimen was glued to a steel plate that was bolted onto the force component transducer. In each test, the shoe was driven forward by the horizontal hydraulic cylinder to contact the floor surface at the heel edge. Another hydraulic cylinder was mounted at the end of the pendulum to simulate the body weight portion supported by the leading foot at heel strike. The two hydraulic cylinders were in a common circuit supplied by a pump that was driven by an electric motor. As the shoe heel passed across the floor surface, the frictional (horizontal: H) and normal (vertical: V) components of the resultant force were measured by the force component transducer.

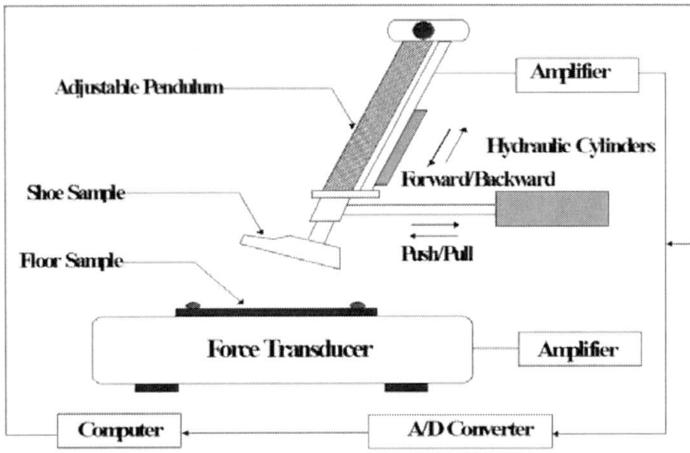

Figure 3.

The test speed was measured by a rotary potentiometer driven by the pendulum shaft. The force component signals and potentiometer voltages were recorded by a desktop computer that continually calculated the H/V force ratio. During the tests, the normal force was maintained around 400 N and the sliding speed was controlled at 40 cm/s based on gait studies (Kim et al., 2013). A heel contact angle of 9° was chosen from the result of previous biomechanical studies (Kim et al., 2013).

Floor and Shoe Specimens

For floor specimens, nine commercially available new flooring specimens were used for the tests. The floor specimens were carefully chosen to include surfaces within a wide range of different surface roughness. Table 1 demonstrates the floor specimens with measured results of the three surface roughness parameters. For shoe specimens, three commercially available new shoes were used for the tests. They included two Nitrile Rubber (S1: Nitrile Rubber No. 1 and S2: Nitrile Rubber No. 2) and a PVC (S3) soles and heels, respectively. The floor and shoe specimens were thoroughly cleaned with demineralized water to eliminate any dirt and dust, and dried and kept in plastic containers during the tests.

Environmental Conditions

Dynamic friction tests were conducted under two different environmental conditions: 1) tap water-covered water wet and 2) soapsuds-covered soapy surface. A commercial type detergent (Kinematic Viscosity: 1.27 *cSt* at 16 °C) was applied to create soapy surface condition. A fixed amount (15 *ml*) of tap water and mixture of water and detergent were sprayed over the whole floor specimen (surface size: 110 × 170 mm) for each environmental condition before the tests. Any debris from the shoe heel was removed using a clean, soft, and dry brush. These procedures are in accordance with parts of BS EN ISO 13287:2012 (International Standard: Personal protective equipment. Footwear. Test method for slip-resistance).

Floor Surface Roughness Measurements

A Talysurf 5 profilometer (Taylor-Hobson, UK) that had a conical stylus with a spherical tip of 12 μm radius was used to measure surface roughness of the floor specimens. To remove waviness components of the surfaces, a Gaussian filter was used with a 0.8 mm cutoff over a single traverse length of 17.5 mm. Surface profiles of each floor specimen were measured five times at three different locations. Measurement results of the surface roughness parameters for each floor specimen were summarized in Table 1.

Table 1. Summary of the floor specimens with surface roughness parameters - *Ra*, *Rt*, and *Rtm*

Floor surface name	Surface roughness Parameter (μm)		
	Ra[a)]	*Rt*[b)]	*Rtm*[c)]
Terrazzo	0.96	8.23	4.85
Smooth Vinyl Tile	1.55	13.61	10.26
Smooth Metal Plate	2.36	13.38	11.76
Smooth Ceramic Tile	3.43	27.50	17.29
Smooth Concrete Slab	6.59	54.00	35.80
Moderate Rough Ceramic Tile	14.54	85.51	61.75
Moderate Rough Concrete Slab	32.97	337.00	224.33
Rough Concrete Slab	44.11	226.75	159.25
Rough Ceramic Tile	70.94	396.80	141.00

a) *Ra* = Center Line Average. b) *Rt* = Maximum Peak-to-Valley Height.
c) *Rtm* = Maximum Mean Peak-to-Valley Height.

Statistical Analysis and Design

Three-way analysis of variance (ANOVA) was performed to determine the significant effects of floor, shoe and environment variables and their interactions on the DFCs. Polynomial regression models were used to evaluate the relationships between the floor surface roughness parameters and DFCs. Independent variables for the ANOVA included the following items:

1) the shoe type ("Shoe") classified by sole/heel materials including two Nitrile Rubber (S1 and S2) and one PVC (S3) heels/soles;
2) the floor type ("Floor") with nine different coarseness defined by surface roughness scales (measured in *Ra*, *Rt*, and *Rtm*); and
3) the walking environment ("Environment") with two different conditions: tap water-covered wet surface and soapsuds-covered soapy surfaces.

The dependent variable for the ANOVA was a dynamic friction coefficient (DFC). A DFC value of 0.4 was used as an acceptable safety criterion to determine the lower bound of the operational range of floor surface roughness. Prevalence odds ratios with a 95% confidence interval were calculated as a measure of association. *P*-values less than 0.05 were considered statistically significant. All statistical analyses were performed using Statistical Analysis System (SAS) software.

RESULTS

Slip-Resistance Performance

Figure 4 shows the results of dynamic friction tests between the nine floor specimens and three shoes under two different environmental conditions. The DFCs were arranged by the order of floor surface roughness, *Ra*.

This arrangement was intended to investigate the relationship between the surface roughness of each floor and DFC results. The DFCs generally increased with the surface roughness of floor specimens and this trend was clearer under the soapy condition than the wet one. However, linear relationships between the surface roughness of floors and DFCs were not found in the case of wet surface condition. Some smooth floors with surface roughness $< 10\ \mu m$ such as smooth vinyl tile, smooth metal plate, and smooth concrete slab showed good slip-resistance performance (DFC > 0.4) against all the shoes (except S2) under the wet condition.

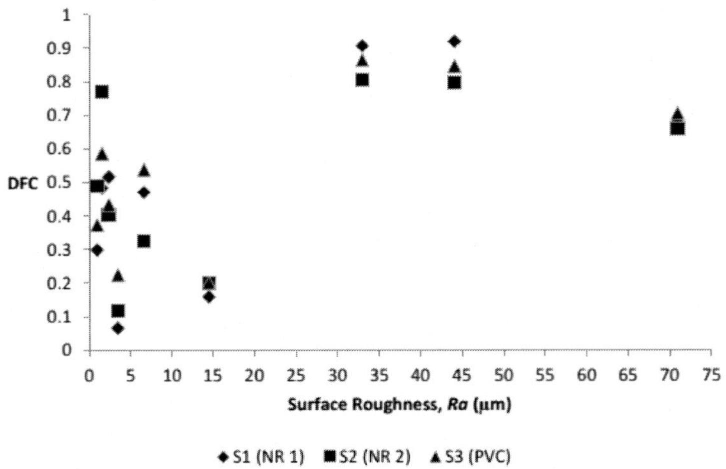

(a) Tap water-covered wet condition

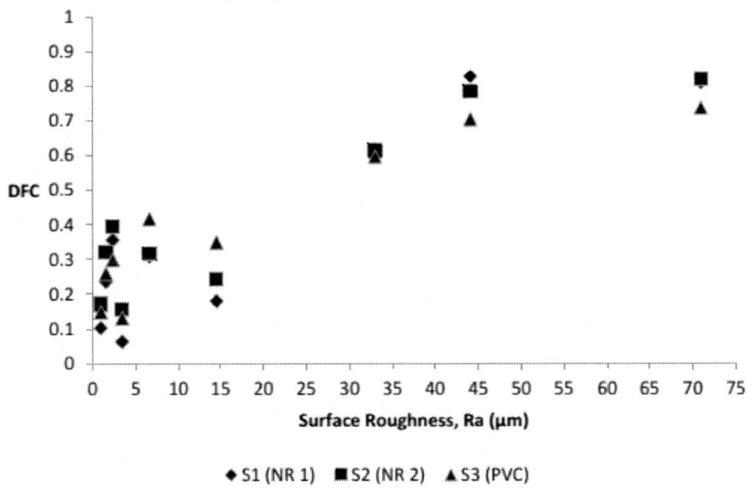

(b) Soapsuds-covered soapy condition

Figure 4.

Interaction between Floor Types and Environments

The three-way ANOVA results (Floor x Shoe x Environment) in Table 2 demonstrate a significant interaction between the Floor (surface roughness) and Environment variables on the DFCs. The DFCs were increased significantly by the floor types with higher surface roughness and drastically reduced under both lubricated surface conditions. However, the effect of floor type was more significant under the soapsuds-covered soapy environment than the tap water-covered wet one. Furthermore, the DFCs under both environments were predicted by cubic functions of three surface roughness parameters: *Ra*, *Rt*, and *Rtm* (see, Table 3). They showed fairly good correlations between the surface roughness parameters of floor specimens and DFC results against each shoe type under both lubricated surface conditions.

Table 2. Summary of three-way analysis of variance (ANOVA) results among the shoes, floors, and environments under the wet and soapy conditions

Effect on DFC	DF	Sum of Squares	Mean Square	F Value	Pr> F
Intercept	1	11.38228	11.38228	4191.25	<.0001
Floor Type [a)]	8	3.02355	0.37794	139.17	<.0001
Environmental Condition	1	0.15424	0.15424	56.8	<.0001
Shoe Type	2	0.00575	0.00288	1.06	0.3699
Floor Type * Environmental Condition	8	0.17495	0.02187	8.05	0.0002
Floor Type * Shoe Type	16	0.11551	0.00722	2.66	0.0294
Environmental Condition * Shoe Type	2	0.00432	0.00216	0.79	0.4689
Error	16	0.04345	0.00272		

a) Floor type as a categorical variable.

Table 3. Regression results: Tap water-covered wet and soapsuds-covered soapy conditions

Environment	Model	DF	R-Square	F Value	Pr> F
Wet	*Ra*	3	0.6428	13.80	<0.0001
	Rt	3	0.6936	17.35	<0.0001
	Rtm	3	0.6995	17.84	<0.0001
Soapy	*Ra*	3	0.8372	39.43	<0.0001
	Rt	3	0.8738	53.07	<0.0001
	Rtm	3	0.8665	49.77	<0.0001

Table 4. Detailed regression analysis results: Tap water-covered wet condition

Roughness Parameters	Variable	DF	Par. Estimate	Standard Error	t value	Pr> |t|
Ra	Intercept	1	0.47596	0.06391	7.45	<0.0001*
	Linear	1	-0.03449	0.01473	-2.34	0.0282*
	Quadratic	1	0.00187	0.00055	3.38	0.0026*
	Cubic	1	-0.00001891	0.00001	-3.7	0.0012*
Rt	Intercept	1	0.50399	0.06462	7.80	<0.0001*
	Linear	1	-0.00663	0.00227	-2.92	0.0078*
	Quadratic	1	0.00006	0.00001	4.01	0.0006*
	Cubic	1	-9.92147E-08	2.34357E-08	-4.23	0.0003*
Rtm	Intercept	1	0.53383	0.06976	7.65	<0.0001*
	Linear	1	-0.01216	0.00402	-3.03	0.0060*
	Quadratic	1	0.00015	0.00004	3.58	0.0016*
	Cubic	1	-4.10128E-07	1.20092E-07	-3.42	0.0024*

* Indicates significant.

Table 5. Detailed regression analysis results: Soapsuds-covered soapy condition

Roughness Parameters	Variable	DF	Par. Estimate	Standard Error	t value	Pr> |t|
Ra	Intercept	1	0.21876	0.04130	5.30	<0.0001*
	Linear	1	0.00264	0.00951	0.28	0.7838
	Quadratic	1	0.00061	0.00036	1.72	0.0990
	Cubic	1	-0.00001	0.00000	-2.45	0.0225*
Rt	Intercept	1	0.23576	0.03970	5.94	<0.0001*
	Linear	1	-0.00081	0.00140	-0.58	0.5684
	Quadratic	1	0.00003	0.00001	2.91	0.0079*
	Cubic	1	-5.31839E-8	1.43968E-8	-3.69	0.0012*
Rtm	Intercept	1	0.23813	0.04449	5.35	<0.0001*
	Linear	1	-0.00139	0.00256	-0.54	0.5940
	Quadratic	1	0.00005	0.00003	1.95	0.0630
	Cubic	1	-1.60083E-7	7.65979E-8	-2.09	0.0479*

* Indicates significant.

Tables 4 and 5 summarize additional statistical information on the regression function parameters for the wet and soapy environments, respectively. They clearly demonstrate the significance of the three roughness parameters on DFCs. The cubic functions of each parameter showed that surface roughness affected DFCs in non-linear fashions and their effects were characterized by three operative zones (Z1: initial low-growth, Z2: steady mid-growth, and Z3: plateau or peak).

Interaction between Shoe Types and Environments

The three-way ANOVA results in Table 2 demonstrated that there were no significant interactions between the Shoe and Environment variables on the DFCs. Some of the shoe types performed better than others, but this effect was evident only for a specific environmental condition. For example, the shoe No. 1 (S1) was better than the shoe Nos. 2 (S2) and 3 (S3) on certain ranges of floor surfaces whilst the shoe No. 3 (S3) was better than the shoe No. 2 (S2) generally under both lubricated environments. However, overall related effects of the shoe type were relatively small as compared to the floor type related ones.

Operational Ranges of Floor Surface Roughness

Figure 5 shows that most of the floor types demonstrate high slip-resistance properties (DFC > 0.4) under the wet environment. However, most of the DFCs were largely decreased and recorded dangerously low levels (DFC < 0.4) under the soapy environment. Acceptable slip-resistance performance was demonstrated only by the three floors with surface roughness > 30 μm in *Ra* roughness parameter: the moderate rough concrete slab, rough concrete slab and rough ceramic tile, respectively. As shown in Table 1, the *Rt* and *Rtm* parameters of these three floors also presented correspondingly high roughness scales. However, the coarser floors such as the rough concrete slab (*Ra* = 44.11 μm) and rough ceramic tile (*Ra* = 70.94 μm) did not provide any further increase of DFCs under both polluted environments as compared to the moderate rough concrete slab (*Ra* = 32.97 μm).

Figure 5 also presents the polynomial regression models for *Ra*, *Rt*, and *Rtm* surface roughness parameters with regression lines of the DFCs under both surface conditions. The cubic functions of regression equations demonstrate examples of possible operational relationships between the floor surface roughness parameters and DFCs for the lubricated conditions. Using the regression models and the minimum safety requirement for DFC > 0.4, it could be estimated that the lower bound ranges for floor surface roughness would be at $Ra \cong 17\ \mu m$, $Rt \cong 120\ \mu m$, and $Rtm \cong 75\ \mu m$ for the soapy condition and $Ra \cong 21\ \mu m$, $Rt \cong 130\ \mu m$, and $Rtm \cong 85\ \mu m$ for the wet condition, respectively. The regression curves on Figure 5 also show that with increments of surface roughness the DFCs under both environmental conditions reach maximum or peak levels (Zone 3) after certain surface roughness scales. From the regression models, it could be estimated that the upper bound ranges for floor surface roughness would be at $Ra \cong 52$ μm, $Rt \cong 300$ μm, and $Rtm \cong 180$ μm, respectively.

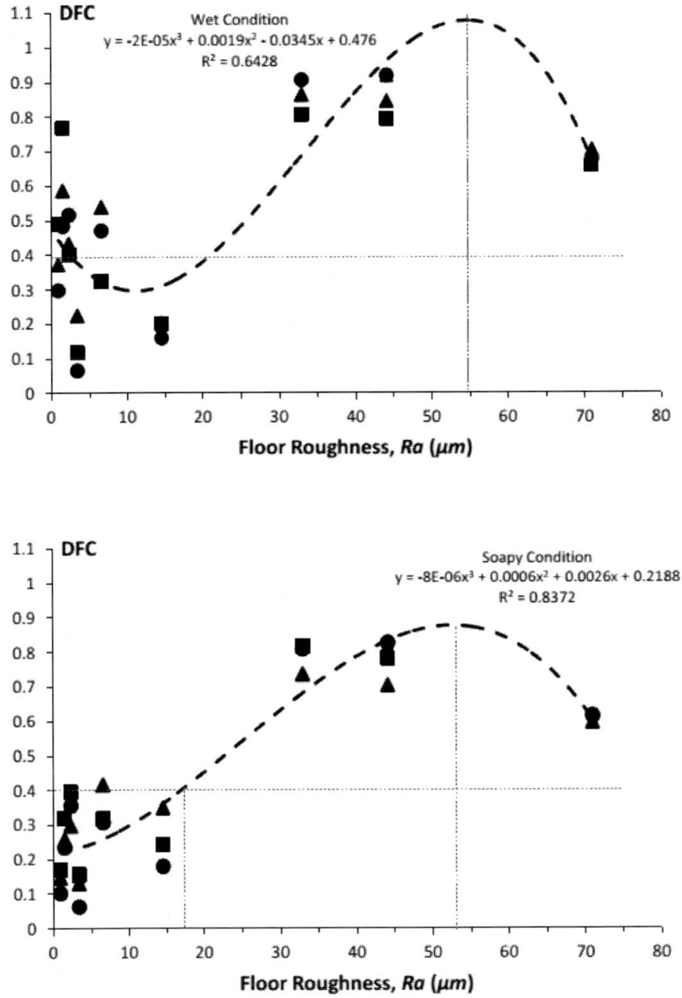

(a) Floor surfce roughness parameter, *Ra* vs. DFCs

Figure 5. (Continued).

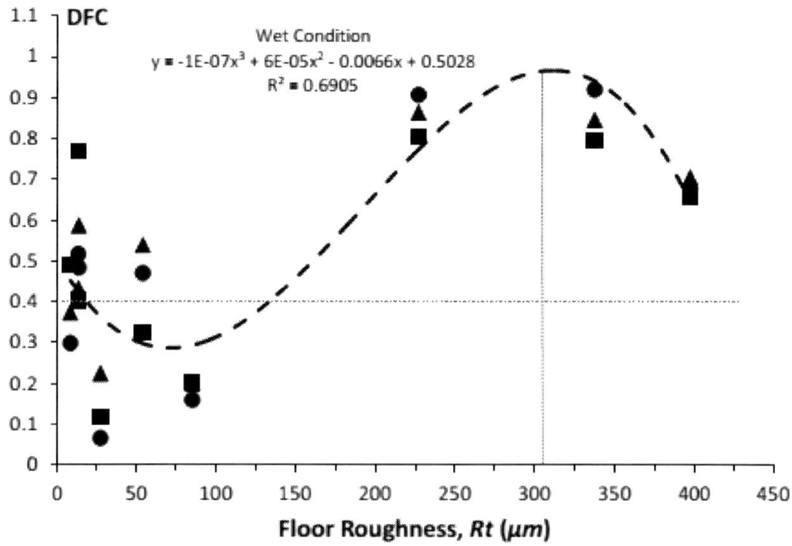

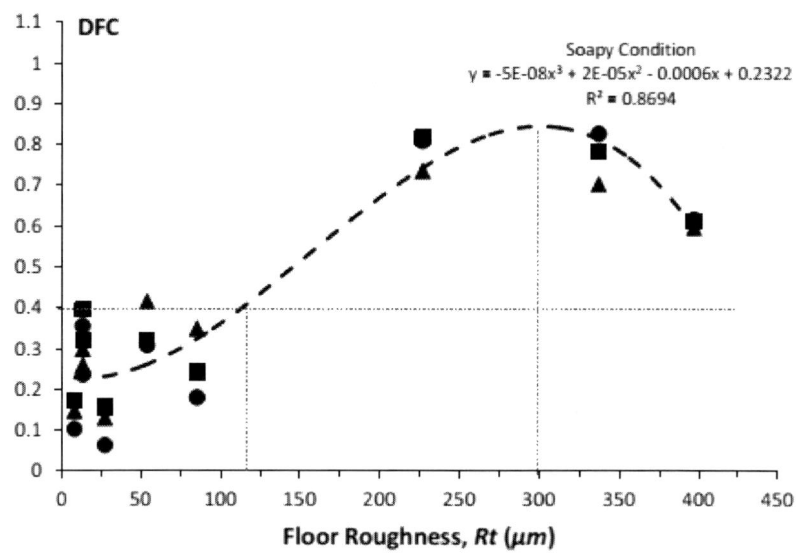

(b) Floor surfce roughness parameter, *Rt* vs. DFCs

Figure 5. (Continued).

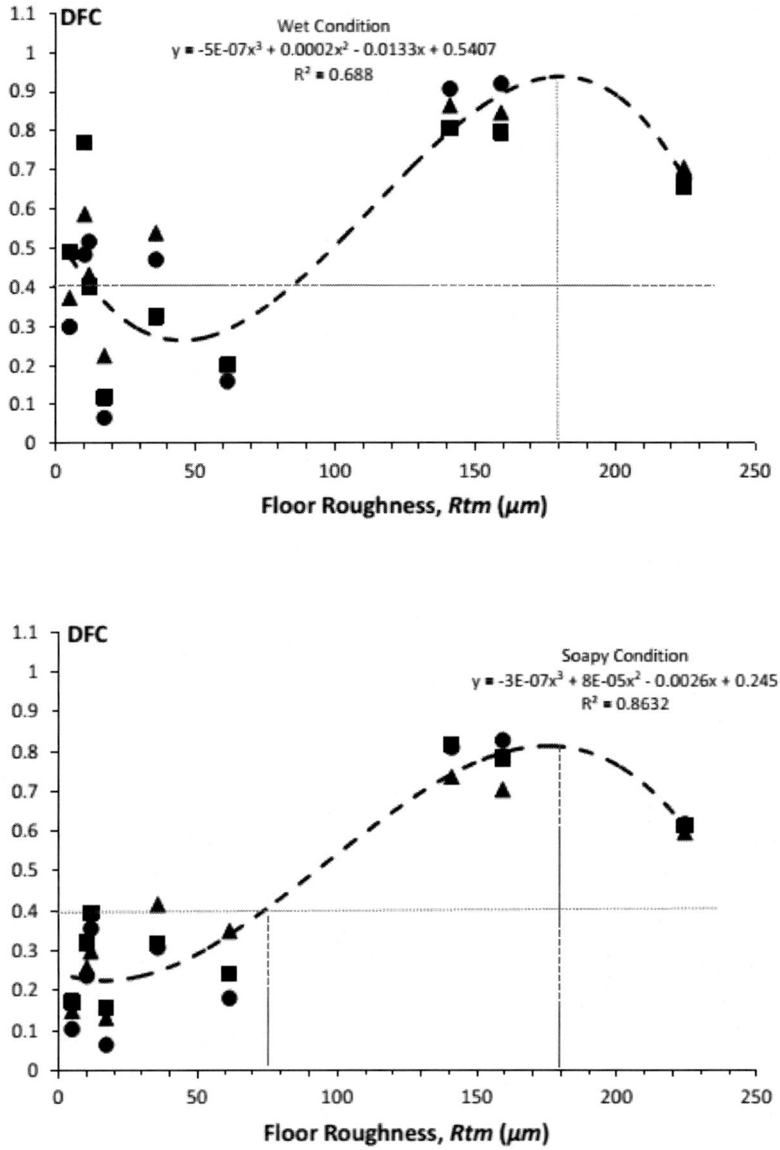

(c) Floor surfce roughness parameter, *Rtm* vs. DFCs

• S1 ■ S2 ▲ S3 - - - - Regression line

Figure 5.

Some of the smooth floor specimens such as smooth vinyl tile (*Ra* = 1.55 μm), smooth metal plate (*Ra* = 2.36 μm), and smooth concrete slab (*Ra* = 6.59 μm) showed relatively good slip-resistance performance under the wet surface condition. But, their slip-resistance properties were dangerously low under the soapy surface condition, thus should not represent an exception from the suggested operational range for the floor surfaces. This slip resistance aspect interfered to estimate the lower bound ranges for floor surface roughness under the wet surface condition.

DISCUSSION

Interaction between Floor Types and Environments

There were significant correlations between the floor types and DFCs under both lubricated conditions. The test results from this chapter clearly supported the main hypothesis from this chapter on the role of floor surface finishes for slip-resistance performance. When the floor surfaces were contaminated, the effect of surface roughness was significant to increase slip-resistance. This outcome was evident in the case of soapsuds-covered soapy surfaces. As shown in Figure 5, there were large increases in the DFCs as the floor surface roughness was increased from 14.54 to 32.97 μm in *Ra* roughness parameter. This increment was even sufficient enough to raise the slip-resistance under the soapy surfaces from a dangerously low level to marginally safe one in DFCs. However, further increments of the floor surface roughness did not provide additional benefits in the slip-resistance performance under both lubricated conditions. This result is consistent with previous studies reporting operational relationships between the surface roughness and DFCs under contaminated conditions (Chang, 2001 & 2002; Manning and Jones, 2001; Kim et al., 2013). It is also found that there is a lack of correlation between the floor-types and DFCs under the wet condition. This finding indicates involvement of multiple mechanisms of slip-resistance properties and possible effects of other tribo-physical characteristics such as hydrodynamic and boundary lubrication effects, and wear developments amongst the floor surfaces, shoe heels, and water wet surfaces during the dynamic friction tests. This aspect requires further studies to understand its complex mechanisms and effects on slip-resistance performance.

Interaction between Shoe Types and Environments

The interaction between the shoe types and environmental conditions demonstrates the importance of shoe selection to improve slip-resistance under the lubricated surfaces. The results in this study suggest that the PVC shoe seems to be a moderate choice for slip-resistance under both contaminated conditions. However, the overall effects of shoe types were relatively small as compared to the floor type effects. This finding suggests that modification of the floor surface would be a more effective strategy to reduce the risks of slip and fall incidents under such polluted environments.

Operational Levels of Floor Surface Roughness

Slip resistance test results from this chapter disclose that increasing the floor surface roughness beyond certain levels does not provide further advantages to enhancing slip-resistance performance. This finding indicates that there exists an operational range of floor surface finishes for optimal slip-resistance functioning. For example, the estimated results suggest that surface roughness in the range of 17 to 52 μm (*Ra* roughness parameter) would be the most effective (DFC > 0.4) for slip-resistant performance under the soapsuds-covered soapy environment. On the other hand, it is interesting to note that the upper bound of floor surface roughness shows similar ranges of surface roughness: 52 μm in *Ra*, 300 μm in *Rt*, and 180 μm in *Rtm* roughness parameters, respectively under both lubricated conditions. As discussed by Kim et al. (2013), there is no study found on a concept of upper bound of floor surface roughness and its operational ranges for safe slip-resistance controls. The present chapter adopted the criteria of "no further benefit for DFC values" to determine the upper boundary of floor surface roughness for slip-resistance performance. Other cut-off criteria to determine the upper boundary of floor surface roughness could be derived from the requirement of safe and comfortable ambulation to avoid falling, but the associated critical DFC values that could be used for such criteria have not been recognized yet. The other issue to be considered would be dealing with developments of wear and tear process of floor surfaces with their long term usages. With continued ambulation, the floor finishes will be continuously modified by wear progression and accordingly operational ranges of floor surfaces will be shifted from optimal ones. However, findings from this chapter confirms that we do not always need to choose rougher floors and/or treat floor surfaces to roughening, which may have important practical design implications as reported in a recent study (Kim et al., 2013).

Limitations of the Current Study

This study tested a small selection of floor specimens with a limited range of surface roughness scales. Further research on the slip-resistance properties of floors and floor coverings with different material and topographic characteristics is required to more precisely determine the specific operational levels of surface roughness. The experimental design of this study also involved only two different lubricated conditions such as water-covered wet and soapsuds-covered soapy surfaces. This limits the applicability of findings only to these types of surface contaminants. Other types of surface pollutants with different compositions and viscosities may result in different operational levels of surface roughness. Studies on a range of shoe types and floor specimens under a range of slippery conditions are in progress.

Conclusion

This study aimed to identify operational ranges of floor surface roughness for effective control of slip resistance performance under two different lubricated environments: tap water-covered wet and soapsuds-covered soapy surfaces from a practical design point for the prevention of walkway slipperiness. The study results showed that all the tested floor-shoe combinations provided insufficient slip-resistance performance under both lubricated surface conditions. Although there were lack of correlations between the surface roughness and DFCs under the wet environment, slip-resistance performance was significantly affected by and well correlated with the floor surface roughness under the soapy one.

Polynomial regression models for the floor surface roughness and DFC relationships allowed estimation of operational ranges of floor surface roughness for optimal slip-resistance performance. Floor surfaces with around 17 μm and 52 μm in *Ra* roughness parameter most likely represent the lower and upper bounds of operational ranges for the most effective control of slip-resistance performance under the soapsuds-covered soapy environment. Findings from this chapter suggest that the proposed concept on operational ranges with lower and upper bounds for the floor surface roughness may have applicable design implications for floors and floor coverings to reduce slip and fall hazards.

ACKNOWLEDGMENTS

The author would like to thank Tsui-Ying Kau from the Clinical Information and Decision Support Services in the University of Michigan Health System at the University of Michigan for her statistical analyses and suggestions to preparing this manuscript.

REFERENCES

AS/NZS 4663. (2004). Slip Resistance Measurements of Existing Pedestrian Surfaces. *Australian Standards AS/NZS 4663*.

Bewoor, A.K., & Kulkarni, V.A. (2009). Metrology & Measurement. Tata McGraw-Hill Education.

British Standards Institution (BSI). (1988). Assessment of Surface Texture, Part 1. Methods and Instrumentation. *BS 1134*, London, UK: British Standards Institution.

Chaffin, D.B., Woldstad, J.C., & Trujillo, M. (1992). Floor/shoe slip resistance measurement. *American Industrial Hygiene Association Journal*, *53*, 283-289.

Chang, W.R. (2001). The effects of surface roughness and contaminant on the dynamic friction of porcelain tile. *Applied Ergonomics*, *32*, 173-84.

Chang, W.R. (2002). The effects of surface roughness and contaminants on the dynamic friction between porcelain tile and vulcanized rubber. *Safety Science*, *40*, 577-91.

Chang, W.R., Kim, I.J., Manning, D.P., &Bunterngchit, Y. (2001). The role of surface roughness in the measurement of slipperiness. *Ergonomics*, *44*, 1200-16.

Derler, S., Kausch, F., and Huber, R. (2008), "Analysis of factors influencing the friction coefficients of shoe sole materials," *Safety Science*, *46*, 822-832.

Harris, G.W., & Shaw, S.R. (1988). Slip resistance of floors: users' opinions, Tortus instrument readings and roughness measurement. *Journal of Occupational Accidents*, *9*, 287-298.

International Organization for Standardization (ISO). (1998). Geometrical Product Specifications (GPS) - Surface Texture: Profile Method - Terms, Definitions and Surface Texture Parameters. ISO 4287: 1997. *International Organization of Standardization*, Switzerland.

Kelsey J. L., Procter-Gray E., Hannan M. T., & Li W. J. (2012). Heterogeneity of falls among older adults: implications for public health prevention. *American Journal of Public Health*, *102*, 2149-2156.

Kim, I.J. (2004a). Development of a new analyzing model for quantifying pedestrian slip resistance characteristics: Part I. Basic concepts and theories. *International Journal of Industrial Ergonomic*, *33*, 395-401.

Kim, I.J. (2004b). Development of a new analyzing model for quantifying pedestrian slip resistance characteristics: Part II. Experiments and validations. *International Journal of Industrial Ergonomics*, *33*, 403-414.

Kim, I.J. (2006a). The current hiatus in fall safety measures, *International Encyclopedia of Ergonomics and Human Factors-2005*. Taylor & Francis Group, LLC, FL., USA, 2563-2567.

Kim, I.J. (2006b). A new paradigm for characterizing slip resistance properties. *International Encyclopedia of Ergonomics and Human Factors-2005*, Taylor & Francis Group, LLC, FL., USA, 2727-2732.

Kim, I.J. (2015). Wear observation of shoe surfaces: Application for slip and fall safety assessments. *Tribology Transactions*, *58*, 407-417.

Kim, I.J., & Smith, R. (2000). Observation of the floor surface topography changes in pedestrian slip resistance measurements. *International Journal of Industrial Ergonomics*, *6*, 581-601.

Kim, I.J., & Smith, R. (2003). A critical analysis of the relationship between shoe-floor wear and pedestrian/walkway slip resistance. In: Marpet, M. and Sapienza, M. editors. *Metrology of Pedestrian Locomotion and Slip Resistance*. American Society of Testing and Materials, Special Technical Publication 1424, ASTM International, Philadelphia. 33-48,

Kim, I.J., & Nagata, H. (2008a). Nature of the shoe wear: Its uniqueness, complexity and effects on slip resistance properties. Contemporary Ergonomics 2008, Taylor & Francis, 728-734.

Kim, I.J., & Nagata, H. (2008b). Research on slip resistance measurements - A new challenge. *Industrial Health*, *46*, 68-78.

Kim, I.J., Smith, R., & Nagata, H. (2001). Microscopic observations of the progressive wear on the shoe surfaces that affect the slip resistance characteristics. *International Journal of Industrial Ergonomics*, *28*, 17-29.

Kim, I.J., Hsiao, H., & Simeonov, P. (2013). Functional levels of floor surface roughness for the prevention of slips and falls: Clean-and-dry and soapsuds-covered wet surfaces. *Applied Ergonomics*, *44*, 58-64.

Leclercq, S., & Saulnier, H. (2002). Floor slip resistance changes in food sector workshops: prevailing role played by 'fouling'. *Safety Science*, *40*, 659-673.

Li, K.W., Chang, W.R., Leamon, T.B., & Chen, C.J. (2004). Floor slipperiness measurement: friction coefficient, roughness of floors, and subjective perception under spillage conditions. *Safety Science*, *42*, 547-565.

Manning, D.P., & Jones, C. (1994). The superior slip-resistance of footwear soling compound T66/103. *Safety Science*, *18*, 45-60.

Manning, D.P., & Jones, C. (2001). The effect of roughness, floor polish, water, oil and ice on underfoot friction: current safety footwear solings are less slip resistant than microcellular polyurethane. *Applied Ergonomics*, *32*, 185-96.

Proctor, T.D. (1993). Slipping accidents in Great Britain - an update. *Safety Science*, *16*, 367-377.

Thomas, T.R. (1999). Rough Surfaces, Second Edition. Imperial College Press, London

Yeoh, H.T., Lockhart, T.E., & Wu, X. (2013). Non-fatal occupational falls on the same level. *Ergonomics*, *56*, 153-65.

In: Accidental Falls
Editor: Brenda Evans

ISBN: 978-1-63483-228-1

Chapter 6

SLIP-RESISTANCE MEASUREMENTS FOR ASSESSING PEDESTRIAN FALL INCIDENTS: FACTS AND FALLACIES

In-Ju Kim
Department of Industrial Engineering, College of Engineering
King Saud University, Riyadh, Saudi Arabia

ABSTRACT

Pedestrian falls resulting from slips and/or trips are one of the leading categories of non-traffic incidents in terms of serious injuries and fatalities. They are a primary cause of industry injuries, as well as one of the leading causes of injury-related deaths for the elderly aged 65 and over. Fall incidents involve multi-factors, but have been commonly assessed by slip-resistance measurements as a simplified format of coefficient of friction (COF) quantity amongst shoes, floors and environments. However, slip-resistance properties have unique and specific features to any combination of the shoe, floor and environment. Notwithstanding such complex characteristics, COFs consistently change because slip-resistance properties are inherently noisy and geometric dimensions between the shoes and floors are largely modified during repetitive measurements. Whilst controversies on the friction measurements for the evaluation of slipperiness remain, slip-resistance properties are still commonly measured by COF readings in many studies and practices for slip and fall safety assessments. To enhance the validity and reliability of friction measurements, therefore, it is necessary to improve our understanding on the slip-resistance mechanics, mechanisms, and related tribo-physical characteristics of the sliding interface amongst the shoes, floors and environments. Because surface topographies of the shoes and floors are largely modified throughout the course of ambulation, this may considerably affect friction and wear behaviours and be one of the most important factors on the slip-resistance properties. Furthermore, surface features significantly affect the degree of slip-resistance performance and have a direct correlation to the ease of cleaning. A high profile surface finish is hard to clean and eventually loses its texture due to inability to remove dirt and physical erosions of the floor surface. This will also increase the risk of slipperiness. However, these issues are hardly investigated in the literature. This study explores the current knowledge gaps and misinterpretations on slip-resistance measurements that are mainly caused by oversimplified perceptions on friction phenomena between the shoes and floors and suggests a new paradigm on slip-resistance assessments for future researches on pedestrian fall incidents.

Keywords: COF, floors, friction, shoes, slip-resistance, tribo-physical characteristics

INTRODUCTION

Slip and fall incidents are one of the most common injuries at work. On average, they cause 40% of all reported major injuries and lead to other types of serious incidents, for example falls from height (HSE, 2011). Slip and fall incidents also have been recognized as a major threat to the safety of individuals not only in industry but also in daily living (Yoon, & Lockhart, 2006). Adults over the age of 70 years have higher mortality rates due to falls than younger people and the increasing incidence of fatality with advancing age is evidenced worldwide (Scott, 2009; Yeoh et al., 2013). According to the World Health Organization, approximately 28-35% of people aged 65 and over fall every year, increasing to 32-42% for those over 70 years of age (WHO, 2007).

Importance of the incident has been recognized due to the magnitude of the problems and associated costs. There have been prolonged efforts to understand the main causes of such incidents in order to reduce their frequency and severity throughout the world. It has been found that the most common precipitating event leading to a fall is a loss of traction or slip-resistance between the shoe sole/heel and floor surface. Its slip-resistance property has been commonly measured as a form of coefficient of friction (COF) (Cohen and Compton, 1982; Harris and Shaw, 1988; Proctor and Coleman 1988; Chaffin et al., 1992; Kim and Smith, 2000 & 2003; Kim et al., 2001; Kim, 2006a & b; Kim and Nagata, 2008a & b). Thus, knowledge about friction demand and friction available has been recognized as a key factor for the fall safety evaluation. Since the COF measurements amongst the shoes, floors and environments were adopted to determine whether a slip was to occur, there have been large disagreements in the interpretation of the results. Importantly, its measurements, analyses, and interpretations have been misguided in many researches and practices for fall safety assessments.

Although the concept of friction is relatively simple and straightforward, solving the real-world problems on slip and fall incidents are a quite complex and challenging task. However, one of the most crucial aspects to address is that the COF is not a constant quantity because initial surface features and topographic characteristics of both shoes and floors are frequently and significantly modified from a first moment of contact by repetitive friction and wear developments. As a result, friction properties become noisy and continuously change as a function of a complex array of tribo-physical phenomena amongst the shoes, floors, and environments (Kim and Smith, 2000 & 2003).

Surprisingly, however, there are little studies on how friction induced wear developments of the shoe heels and floor surfaces affect the slip-resistance performance. In addition, slip-resistance properties observed at the sliding interface between the shoe heel and floor surface are diverse and combine various sub-mechanisms of friction and wear events (Kim and Smith, 2000 & 2003; Kim, 2004a). Thus, a simple format of friction measurement does not provide an accurate determination of essential properties of slip-resistance between the shoes and floors and accordingly has obvious difficulty as an indicator for the fall safety measures.

In this sense, a fresh insight would be required to systematically approach multiple characteristics of friction and wear behaviours between the shoes and floors and their interactions to better feature the slip-resistance properties than a commonly practiced mean or averaged COF reading. Whilst controversies around the friction measurement for slipperiness assessment still remain (Chang et al., 2001; Kim, 2004a & b; Kim and Nagata, 2008a & b), a tribo-physical approach may provide an objective alternative to overcome the current limitations on slip-resistance evaluations. Therefore, this chapter robustly discussed the limitations and mislead concepts on slip-resistance measurements and analysed the seriousness of misinterpretations on slip-resistance properties that were mainly caused by oversimplified conceptions on friction phenomena between the shoe heels and floor surfaces. Based on those critical analyses, a new paradigm on friction and wear behaviours between the shoes and floors was proposed for the future researches on slip-resistance measurements.

BASIC QUESTIONS AND FALLCIES

A great deal of research has been undertaken for the prevention of pedestrian slip and fall incidents. Many different theories, devices and experiments have been developed to establish safety criteria in terms of static friction coefficient (SFC) as well as dynamic friction coefficient (DFC), or slip-resistance properties amongst the shoe-floor-environment combinations (Kim and Smith, 2003). As a result, most studies from a variety of slip-resistance testers and apparatuses have referenced their own COF indices as a safety threshold for slip risk assessment. However, this approach seems to have serious limitations. Because each testing device or tool has different theoretical concepts and technical principles, it would be unreasonable to adopt the reference COF value without any citation to the instrument employed for the slip-resistance measurements. This means that there is a great uncertainty about what a "safe" index for the COF between the footwear and underfoot surface should be.

Another critical aspect to highlight is that the COF index or quantity is not a constant value and continuously changes (Kim et al., 1998; Kim and Smith, 2000; Kim et al., 2013; Kim, 2015). Because topographic characteristics of both shoe and floor surfaces are continuously varied through the course of combined effect of friction and wear developments. That is, initial surface features and topographic structures are significantly altered and continuously modified from the first moment of contact by surface failures and wear progresses (Proctor and Coleman, 1988; Kim and Smith, 2000 & 2003; Kim et al., 2001; Kim, 2004a; Kim and Nagata, 2008; Kim et al., 2013; Kim, 2015). In addition, friction phenomena observed at a sliding interface between any footwear and floor surface are diverse and combine various sub-mechanics and mechanisms (Leclercq et al., 1993; Grönqvist, 1995; Kim and Smith, 2000 & 2003; Kim et al., 2013; Kim, 2015). Therefore, a simple format of friction measurement may not be accurate enough to provide a true measure of slip-resistance properties between the footwear and underfoot surface. In spite of the importance of those complex issues, this matter has not been systematically analysed in the literature yet. Hence, it would be beneficial to review the definition of friction and redefine it from a fresh point of view.

DEFINITION OF A COF

As a well-known quantity, a coefficient of friction (COF) has long been used as a fall safety indicator or index. It is easy to define, but hard to understand its overall characteristics. Traditionally, friction is defined as the force resistance to relative motion developed between two bodies in contact with one another, or more comprehensively, as the latent resistive force which opposes incipient movement at and parallel to the slip plane of two interfacing surfaces (Ludema, 1987). Characterization of the relative magnitude of this force is done most conveniently by expressing it as the ratio of the force required to just overcome the resisting force to the force acting perpendicular to the two surfaces in contact. That is, a COF is a property of the two interfacing and interacting surfaces and serves as a measure of their micro- and macro-roughness, inter- and intra-molecular forces of attraction and repulsion, and their viscoelastic (polymer and/or elastomer deformation) properties (Miller, 1983). As such, surface topographies of both bodies, contact areas, contact time, velocity of movement, pressure, and material types are major contributing factors to the COF results. The COF is also referred to as either static (SFC) or dynamic (or kinetic) friction coefficient (DFC) depending on whether it is a measure of the forces at the instant relative motion begins or after there is a continuous, uniform sliding motion, respectively (Moore, 1972 & 1975).

Because of the complex nature and multi-factors involved, the measured COF quantities seem to show inconsistencies even as the same shoe-floor combinations are employed for assessing their slip-resistance performance. This reality has been recognized as a great concern when different friction testers, sensors and/or protocols are adopted to measure slip-resistance performance in the literature (Kim, 2004a). However, most slip safety measures and assessments have simply reported that a particular shoe or floor surface resists the movement of a particular floor surface or one's shoe sole across its surface. Wherein co-equal contributions of the footwear or floor surface is either ignored or not even considered. As addressed in the above, a COF quantity is not a constant for any particular material, but is typical of two bodies sliding against each other under a given set of environmental conditions. Therefore, any question of either "what is a COF of this floor or floor covering?" or "what is a COF of that shoe?" would be an unreasonable enquiry. The question should be raised by either "what type of shoes was measured or tested against which floor surfaces?" or "what is a COF index or quantity between this shoe and that floor surface?"

AVERAGE OR MEDIAN COF

One of the key issues challenged from slip-resistance measurements seems to not only a simple matter of friction measurement but also a primary aspect of friction mechanics and mechanisms between the shoes and floors. This means that an average or median COF index is likely to be a quite controversial issue to confine a slip-resistance property between the shoe and floor. This seems to oversimplify the multifaceted nature of tribo-physical phenomena observed at the sliding interfaces amongst the shoes, floors and environments. Figure 1 shows a simple example of slip-resistance measurements between a PVC shoe and a smooth vinyl floor as a function of test times under clean and dry surface conditions.

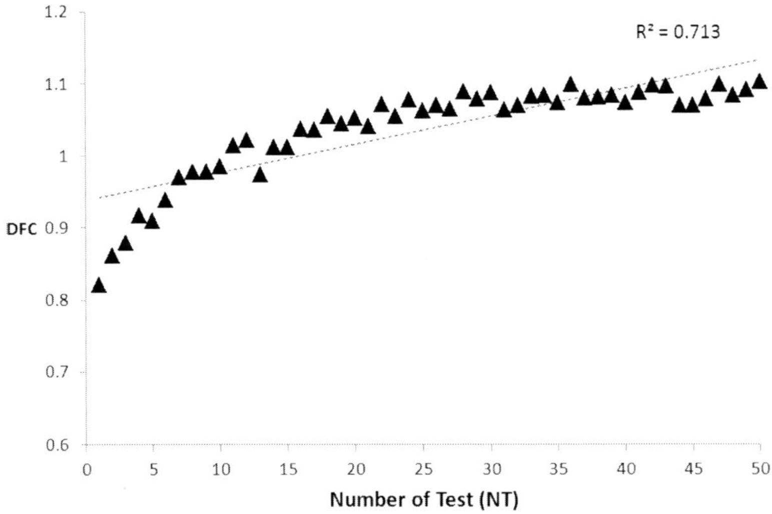

Figure 1.

As shown in Figure 1, the DFCs were gradually increased from 0.821 to 1.070 after the test. For a detailed investigation, the DFC results were divided into five stages. Each stage was counted on the basis of ten times of rubbings. When compared the DFC results between the stage Nos. 1 and 5, there were clear differences in their slip-resistance performance despite a limited of rubbings. From the DFC results, the following questions are challenged:

1. How can define a DFC quantity (or value) for this combination of the PVC shoe and vinyl floor?

As summarized in Table 1, statistical results show evident comparisons in each test stage. In this condition, it is not clear what DFC quantity should be used for rating slip-resistance performance between the PVC shoe and vinyl floor.

Table 1. Basic statistical descriptions on the DFC results between a PVC shoe and a smooth vinyl floor after 50 times of dynamic friction tests

Basic Statistics	DFC Results				
	Stage 1	Stage 2	Stage 3	Stage 4	Stage 5
Minimum	0.821	0.973	1.040	1.063	1.070
Maximum	0.985	1.054	1.089	1.098	1.102
Mean	0.924	1.025	1.069	1.079	1.087
Standard Deviation	0.057	0.024	0.015	0.010	0.012
R-Square	0.935	0.570	0.585	0.138	0.037

2. How many test numbers are required for a valid and reliable DFC quantity?

Because the measured DFC results between the PVC shoe and vinyl floor continuously change during the test, it is very difficult to reach a decision on a number of test rubbings for achieving reliable test results. DFCs seem to highly dependent upon the test conditions of both bodies such as number of rubbings and service records of both shoes and floors.

3. What is a reliably representing DFC quantity?

As shown in the test, it is strongly questioned that what a representative DFC index (or value) is for this case. Should we choose 0.924 from stage 1 or 1.070 from stage 5 or a mean of stages 1 to 5 or need more tests?

The above mentioned questions are not only a matter of the current dilemmas on slip-resistance measurements, but also a matter of primal issues for the requirement of in-depth understanding on friction and wear phenomena amongst the shoes, floors and environments. Therefore, it is urged that the simplified concept of average or median COF readings for slip-resistance assessments needs thorough investigations.

WEAR DEVELOPMENTS

Wear developments between the shoe heel/sole and floor surface seems to be a major concern and considerably affect slip-resistance properties. Wear behaviours are the results of many local events and the nature of these phenomena are very difficult to determine unless analyze them at a very early stage of slip-resistance measurements. The physical, chemical, and mechanical properties in surface and near-surface regions may well differ from the corresponding bulk properties of the materials. These surface and near-surface regions can change radically as a result of interaction of the surface molecules with their environments and with each other throughout the course of repetitive friction and wear processes. As a result, slip-resistance is neither a constant nor an intrinsic property of any particular material compositions, but changes constantly. Hence, initial and rubbed surfaces of shoes and floors need to be quantitatively and qualitatively analyzed to assess and explore wear behaviours.

Questions related to shoe and floor wear behaviours are only found in few of the recent studies (Manning, et al., 1998; Kim and Smith, 2000 & 2003; Kim, et al., 2001; Kim and Nagata, 2008a; Kim, 2015). These studies reported that the surface topographies of the shoes and floor constantly changed in specific ways during slip-resistance measurements. For example, extended rubbings on the shoe heels caused structural changes to the initial surfaces and to the COFs. Menezes, et al. (2009) also conducted experiments to understand the role of surface texture and roughness parameters on the COFs and transfer layer formation.

Although those studies showed strong relationships between the surface roughness and slip-resistance properties, essential understandings on tribo-physical characteristics for wear mechanics and mechanisms of the shoe and floor surfaces were not fully explored. In particular, there are no definitive concepts and methodical studies on the wear behaviours of shoe and floor surfaces. It is considered that observations of wear-induced topographic changes may suggest a possible new design idea for shoes and floors to improve slip-resistance properties.

Despite the importance of this issue, it is hard to find any systematic studies to understand wear development of shoe and floor surfaces and identify their effects on pedestrian walkway slip-resistance performance. Therefore, it is recommended that future researches need to pay attentions on those areas.

MAINTENANCE ISSUES

COFs of textured floors and floor coverings may be quickly lost without effective cleaning procedures and maintenances. The flooring material itself significantly influences the degree of slip-resistance (Murphy, 2003). For example, soft flooring materials such as rubber or urethane are less slippery than hard surfaces such as ceramic or metal. Unfortunately, however, some of the softer materials are not viable for industrial applications. These surfaces generally require an abrasion-resistant surface that can withstand heavy impact and traffic conditions (Murphy, 2003). To accommodate these conditions, most slip-resistant industrial floors are composed of a polymeric material (Shore Hardness D >50) usually incorporating some degree of aggregate (ASTM D 2240).

The porosity of floors will affect the slip-resistance under wet conditions. For example, concrete slabs absorb waters, whilst waters stay on the surface if coated with epoxy. To address this issue, polymeric floors are installed with various surface finishes. This allows waters (or other contaminants) to move out of the way of contacting surfaces. The surface texture or topography can be changed by applying a stipple finish polymer to an aggressive texture using bonded aggregate (Murphy, 2003). Most industrial environments require only a slight non-skid texture to avoid slips and falls. This can be accomplished using a fine aggregate incorporated into the topcoat surface of the floor.

The degree to surface texture has a direct correlation to the ease of cleaning (Gould, 2003). A high profiled or textured floor finish will be hard to clean and eventually lose its surface features due to inability to remove the dirt. Some cleaning materials will also leave residuals that can contribute to the slipperiness of the floor surface. It is best to match the cleaner to the contaminant followed by effective removal of the detergent and contaminants.

All flooring materials gradually wear with use. For example, physical erosions of the floor will polish the surface finishes increasing the risks of slipperiness. Depending upon the materials applied in the floors and floor coverings, this process can be extended greatly. Surface features and finishes will definitely impact on the cleanability of surfaces, but the effect on cleanability and maintenance issues with slip and fall prevention has not yet been studied to any great extent. Therefore, future researches should pay more attentions in those areas as well.

SURFACE ANALYSES

Significance of Surface Analysis

The recent literature reports that surface roughness of the shoes and floors have substantial effects on slip-resistance performance under different types of walking environments (Grönqvist, 1995; Rowland et al., 1996; Wilson, 1996; Manning et al., 1998; Kim and Smith, 2000 & 2003; Kim et al., 2001; Kim, 2004a & 2004b; Kim and Nagata, 2008; Kim et al., 2013; Kim, 2015). Surface roughness provides necessary drainage spaces to avoid squeeze film formations under contaminated environments. Micro- and macro-tread patterns on the shoe heel/sole surface increase slip-resistance properties by providing spaces for the removal of pollutants and lead to an increase in direct contacts with the floor surface. Thus, large-scale roughness and/or tread patterns are commonly designed into the shoe bottom areas, but they quickly become inadequate after being worn. Geometric characteristics of the floor surface, however, could rather drastically improve slip-resistance properties than the shoe cases. Because the floor surfaces may provide shaper, taller, and tougher asperities that would be enough to extend upward through lubricating films sufficiently to engage with the bottom areas of heel surfaces in a manner like sandpapers (Kim and Nagata, 2008). Hence, surface roughness of the shoes and floors should be fully observed with friction and wear measurements when analysing the slip-resistance properties.

Although key theory concepts and model developments to predict slip-resistance properties from known surface characteristics have not reached a mature stage yet, if the surface features of shoes and floors and their interactions could be quantitatively measured and systematically analysed, then our understanding on the multifaceted characteristics of friction and wear behaviours would be considerably enhanced. On a broader scale, this may also assist to improve design aspects of the footwear and floor surfaces that consequently lead to substantial reductions in the slip and fall incidents (Kim, et al., 2013; Kim, 2015).

Major Effects of Surface Roughness

Progressive wear and surface changes of shoe surfaces during slip-resistance measurements were examined by Kim et al. (2001). They showed that variations in the surface geometry of the shoe heels had a major effect on the slip-resistance properties. Kim and Smith (2000 & 2003) also analysed the topography changes of floor surfaces before and after the slip-resistance measurements. This study found that embedding of polymeric materials from shoe heels into the valley areas of floor surfaces was a major cause of the changes of floor surface geometry. Other studies also showed that surface roughness parameters were well correlated with the standard deviation of peak heights and the changes in surface roughness within the contact areas, as well as comparative facing of two surfaces between the shoe heels and floors during the dynamic friction tests (Kim, 2004a & 2004b; Kim and Nagata, 2008a & b). A recent study suggests a theory concept and wear model to explore tribo-physical characteristics of the shoe surfaces and their fundamental aspects on underlying mechanisms of wear behaviours (Kim, 2015).

All those studies clearly identified that surface topographies of the shoes and floors underwent remarkable changes during slip-resistance measurements. As a result, surface changes of the shoes and floors throughout the course of recurring friction and wear developments had a major effect on slip-resistance results. Those studies also found that wear and wear-induced surface alterations and failures were more severe than expected and occurred at a very early stage of dynamic slip-resistance measurements. That is, slip-resistance properties between the shoes and floors depend not just on the friction when a slip starts, but also on how the wear develops as slip progress. Therefore, it becomes evident that surface features of both shoes and floors should be comprehensively analysed with the measurements of slip-resistance properties.

Suggestion of a New Paradigm

Tribo-Physical System

One of the most important characteristics in the shoe-floor tribo-physical system would be a material property of the shoes, where the surface topography rapidly changes and continuously produces wear products during every single rubbing. Because elastic modulus of the shoe soles/heels is considerably lower than that of flooring materials, it could be assumed that wear behaviours mostly occur at the heel contact areas caused by protuberances on the floor surface.

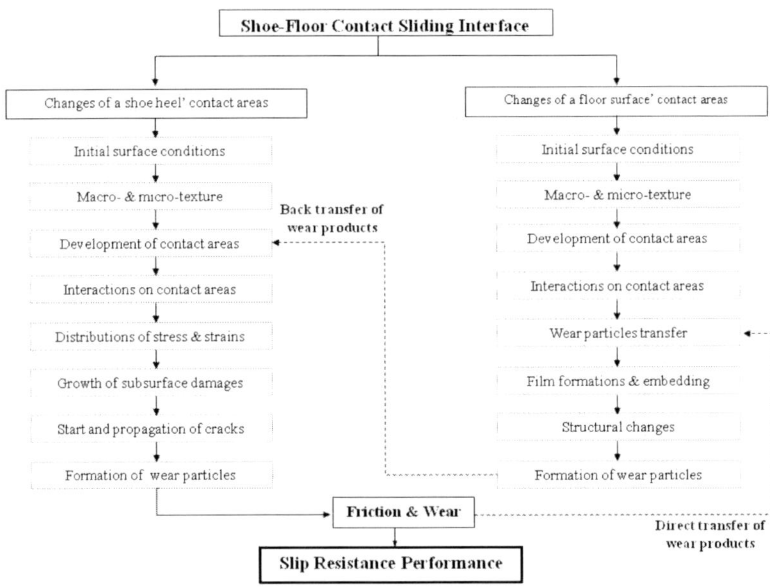

Figure 2.

Figure 2 suggests a schematic diagram for an estimated wear cycle between a shoe heel and floor surface during repetitive ambulation. As shown in Figure 2, the heel surface would be involved into an immediate wear development from an initial contact to particle formations during rubbing events. Since surface changes leading to wear outcomes seem to be largely caused by forces acting on contact areas, macroscopic operating conditions such as tread patterns and shoe material types could not define the process by themselves. On the other hand, specific micro-topographies of the heel surface may determine the contact conditions between the two surfaces under a range of walking conditions. The actual forces working on the contact areas then establish subsurface stress fields and strain distributions, which could result in accumulation of damages eventually leading to removal of wear products. An important point in this process is that the formation of wear particles seems to be accompanied by gradual and/or abrupt changes of topographies in the heel surface. As a result, a feedback loop as shown in Figure 2 would be considered during repetitive rubbings. The worn heel surfaces will affect contact sliding conditions and accordingly slip-resistance results. Hence, micro- and macro-topographies are not a given property, but constantly modified throughout the course of wear evolutions. This seems to cause wide differences in the wear rates often experienced under macroscopically similar type of shoes.

It also could be assumed that relocation of worn materials to its counterface seems to be a crucial characteristic of the wear mechanisms between the floor surface and shoe heel/sole. The formation of wear products such as transferring films and particles on the counterface during repetitive walking plays an important role in the wear and friction mechanisms of materials (Bahadur, 2000; Kim and Nagata, 2008a; Kim, 2015). Thus, the transferred wear products seem to be equally important for the understanding of tribo-physical behaviours between the shoes and floor surfaces. In other words, unlike other mechanical properties, wear properties of the materials are not intrinsic but are instead specific to the sliding system and are modifiable by the sliding variables such as counterface roughness (Bahadur et al., 1996; Yu & Bahadur, 1998; Zhao & Bahadur, 1998 & 1999).

In the shoe-floor sliding friction system, the variables are closely related to the development of wear products so they affect wear resistance of the floor surfaces. Therefore, the issues of wear formations and developments of the floor surface also should be fully explored in the future study.

Model Development for Shoe Wear

Main Hypothesis

When a shoe heel is loaded against a floor, it could be assumed that two surfaces initially touch only at tiny discrete areas where their highest asperities are in contact, as illustrated in Figure 3 (a). A local pressure at the contact regions would be high enough to cause plastic deformations of the heel asperities even at the lightest load because an elastic modulus of the shoe heel would be significantly less than that of the floor surface. Hence, its contact mechanism would be an interlocking status as shown in Figure 3 (b) with a magnified format. If the shoe heel slides on the floor surface, then the heel surface would be ruptured, deformed and ploughed by wedge-shaped asperities of the floor surface (Figure 3 (c)). During this process, the shoe surface seems to be continuously changed and damaged by wear developments. Repetitive rubbings by continuous walking would require hard asperities of the floor surface to plough grooves in the heel surface areas. This cyclic rubbing or walking events, therefore, are likely to contribute to further developments of shoe wear so that wear growth of the heel surface would be unavoidable.

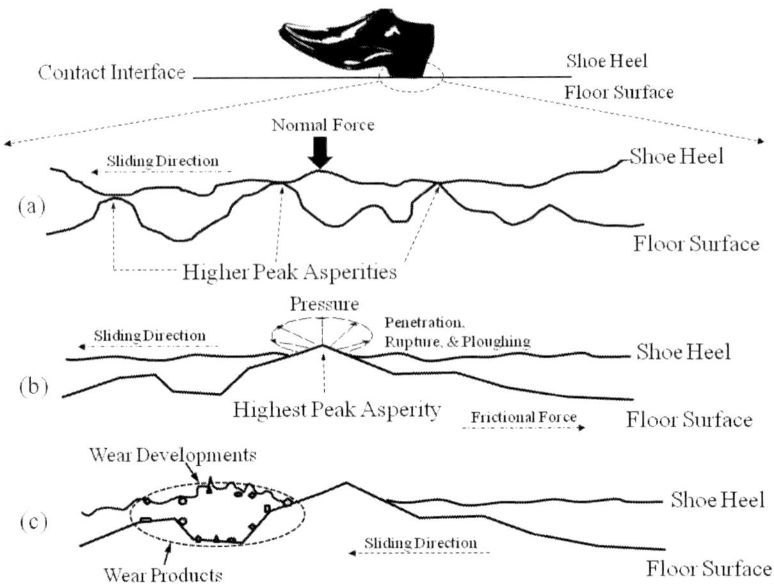

Figure 3.

Shoe Wear Model

Predominant wear types observed at the shoe surface would be primarily subjected to abrasive and adhesive behaviours due to the nature of contact-sliding mechanisms of our walking mode (Kim, 2015). Other types of wear behaviours such as ploughing, material transfer/relocation, and fatigue could be considered. Ploughing could take place when adhesive and abrasive wear do not include any material removal from the heel surface but only relocation of polymeric materials. Subsequent rubbings may eliminate protruding materials by abrasive wear. In this process, material pick-ups or transfers between the shoe heel and floor surface could occur because polymeric materials from the shoe heel could be left inside the floor surface asperities and vice versa. Fatigue wear would be different from the adhesive and abrasive wear behaviours and characterized by formation of large cracks after a critical number of loadings. Prior to this critical point, only negligible wear developments seem to be taking place. Fatigue wear could occur when the heel surfaces are exposed to a large number of alternating tensile and compressive stresses, which are typical modes of heel striking and sliding during our ambulation. Large wear fragments may be formed due to weakening of the underlying layers of heel surfaces. Based on those assumptions, a shoe wear model is suggested in the following:

1. Adhesive wear

Adhesive wear would be taken place when relative movements between the shoe and floor induce breakages of the junction inside the shoe heel rather than at the interface. Adhesive wear will affect only upper layers of the surface, where the tops of asperities will be broken off.

2. Abrasive wear

Abrasive wear would be considered as events by displacement of polymeric materials from the shoe heel in relative sliding motion caused by ploughing effects of hard protuberances on the floor surface, such as peak asperities and/or embedded hard particles. Abrasive wear will affect both upper and lower layers of the heel surface because polymeric materials can be removed from valley areas as well as from peak ones.

3. Ploughing

Ploughing could take place when abrasion does not include any material removal from the heel surface but only relocation of materials. Ploughing will affect both upper and lower layers of the heel surface because polymeric materials will be moved on the surface, forming peaks and leaving valleys.

4. Fatigue wear

Fatigue wear could be occurred when the heel surface is exposed to a large number of alternating tensile and compressive stresses, which are typical modes of heel striking and sliding from walking phases. That is, as the floor surface becomes blunt rather than sharp projections, the heel surface will undergo cyclic deformations, and surface failures due to fatigue wear eventually will occur. Fatigue wear would affect only lower layers of the surface because cracks will start from valley areas and form more valley ones of asperities. Fatigue wear may differ from the above wear mechanisms being characterized by the formation of large cracks after a critical number of repetitive loadings. Prior to this critical point, only minor or negligible wear would be taken place.

Model Development for Floor Wear

Main Hypotheses

Formation of transferring films and wear particles on the counterface seems to play an important role in the wear and friction mechanisms of materials (Bahadur, 2000). Thus, it could be anticipated that the floor surfaces are experienced certain types of wear and surface alterations during the repetitive ambulation. For example, film depositions or transferring of abraded polymer particles from the shoe heel into the floor surface would be one possibility. In this case, material pick-ups would be added to the wear mechanism. The material pick-ups will prevalently affect the upper layer of the floor surface because deposits of polymeric materials will be added to the peak heights. Hence, wear observation should be extended to surface topographies of the floors with measuring their slip resistance properties.

Floor Wear Model

Whilst there is no reliable theory or a model to accurately predict the direction and relative amount of wear transfer for the floor-shoe sliding friction system yet, the simplest hypothesis would be that transfer should occur if the shear strength of adhesive bonds between asperities of two mating surfaces is greater than that of the transferring materials. Thus, one may expect that the softer materials (shoe heels) would be mainly transferred into the harder ones (floor surfaces).

Based on the above assumptions, a floor wear model is suggested in the following three ways:

1) one-way transfer: shoe heels to floor surfaces or floor surfaces to shoe heels
2) back transfer: shoe heels to floor surface & floor surfaces to shoe heels
3) mutual transfer: shoe heels to floor surfaces and floor surface to shoe heels

Figure 4 proposes an integrated wear model for the floor surface rubbed against the shoe heel during sustained pedestrian ambulation. It demonstrates three possible sources of flooring wear mechanisms: direct (one-way), back (two-ways), and mutual (multi-ways) transfer wear modes. It also demonstrates formations and movements of wear products between the floor surface and shoe heel. The wear system between the floor surface and shoe heel/sole seems to have a reciprocal relationship.

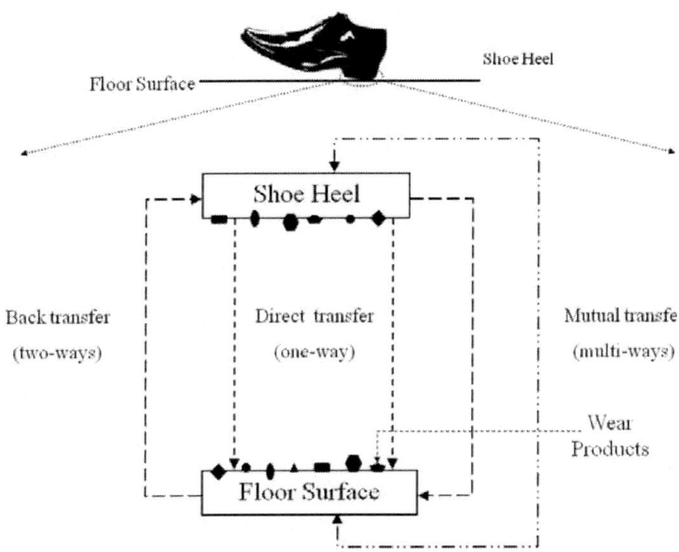

Figure 4.

Conclusion

As clearly addressed in the introduction of this chapter, a simple format of friction measurement may misrepresent the complex nature of slip-resistance properties amongst the shoes, floors, and environments. Facilitated routine friction measurements from laboratory environments also could oversimplify essential aspects of slip-resistance properties. Although there has been considerable research progress on the understanding of slip-resistance properties and its performance, it would be probably true to mention that none of the COF measurements reported to date could be regarded as final objective values for any chosen shoe-floor-environment combination. As long as the controversy around friction measurement as a format of COF index remains, improvements in the principal concepts and methodologies on slip-resistance properties and measurements are urgently required. Therefore, it is essential for researchers working on slip and fall safety to find improved concepts and measurement methods to assess the slipperiness for complementing current activities. This should be based on thorough comprehension on the multifaceted nature of friction and wear phenomena and surface analysis techniques for characterizing the surfaces of shoes and floors and their interactions during slip-resistance measurements.

Potential forms of friction and wear characteristics of the shoes and floors were clearly explored by demonstrating the complexity of mechanics and mechanisms involved. The contribution of surface roughness to slip-resistance is linked to the fundamental knowledge of friction and wear behaviours of the shoes and floors. However, to date these factors have hardly been considered in the slip and fall safety research area. In this context, this chapter was focused on broadening the knowledge base and developing new notions for characterizing the slip-resistance properties from a tribo-physical point of view on which advancements in the validity and reliability of slip-resistance measurements might be made. It is wished that suggestions from this chapter would not only provide a sound theoretical foundation for the understanding of both frictional and wear phenomena between the footwear and underfoot surfaces but also enhance the creditability of overall pedestrian fall safety assessments. Although theoretical model developments for the shoe-floor tribo-physical system have not yet reached a stage where it would be quantitatively possible to predict the slip-resistance property from known tribo-physical characteristics, this new paradigm may provide an insight to identifying the complex issues. Therefore, factoring in wear-induced material changes with friction measurements may provide a way of enhancing the reliability of fall safety determinations over the current methodology for COF readings.

REFERENCES

Bahadur, S. (2000). The development of transfer layers and their role in polymer tribology. *Wear*, *245*, 92-99.

Bahadur, S., Gong, D., & Anderegg, J. (1996). Investigation of the influence of CaS, CaO, and CaF2 fillers on the transfer and wear of nylon by microscopy and XPS analysis. *Wear,* 197, 271-279.

Chaffin, D.B., Woldstad, J.C., & Trujillo, M. (1992). Floor/shoe slip resistance measurement. *American Industrial Hygiene Association Journal*, *53*, 283-289.

Chang, W.R., Grönqvist, R., Leclercq, S., Myung, R., Makkonen, L., Strandberg, L., Brungraber, R.J., Mattke, U., & Thorpe, S.C. (2001). The role of friction in the measurement of slipperiness, Part 1: Friction mechanisms and definition of test conditions. *Ergonomics*, *44*, 1217-1232.

Cohen, H.H., & Compton, D.M.J. (1982). Fall accident patterns: characterization of most frequent work surface-related injuries. *Professional Safety*, 27, 16-22.

Gould, P. (2003). Smart, clean surfaces. *Materials Today*, *6(11)*, 44-48.

Grönqvist, R. (1995). Mechanisms of friction and assessment of slip resistance of new and used footwear soles on contaminated floors. *Ergonomics*, *38*, 224-241.

Harris, G.W., & Shaw, S.R. (1988). Slip resistance of floors: users' opinions, Tortus instrument readings and roughness measurement. *Journal of Occupational Accidents*, *9*, 287-298.

Health and Safety Executive (HSE). 2011. Investigation of slip resistance and the hygienic cleaning of floors in hospital settings. *RR889 Research Report*. Available from: http://www.hse.gov.uk/research/rrpdf/rr889.pdf.

Kim, I.J. (2004a). Development of a new analyzing model for quantifying pedestrian slip resistance characteristics: Part I. Basic concepts and theories. *International Journal of Industrial Ergonomic*, *33*, 395-401.

Kim, I.J. (2004b). Development of a new analyzing model for quantifying pedestrian slip resistance characteristics: Part II. Experiments and validations. *International Journal of Industrial Ergonomics*, *33*, 403-414.

Kim, I.J. (2006a). The current hiatus in fall safety measures. *International Encyclopedia of Ergonomics and Human Factors-2005*, Taylor & Francis Group, LLC, FL., USA, 2563-2567.

Kim, I.J. (2006b). A new paradigm for characterizing slip resistance properties. *International Encyclopedia of Ergonomics and Human Factors-2005*, Taylor & Francis Group, LLC, FL., USA, 2727-2732.

Kim, I.J. (2015). Wear observation of shoe surfaces: Application for slip and fall safety assessments. *Tribology Transactions*, *58*, 407-417.

Kim, I.J., & Smith, R. (2000). Observation of the floor surface topography changes in pedestrian slip resistance measurements. *International Journal of Industrial Ergonomics*, *6*, 581-601.

Kim, I.J., & Smith, R. (2003). A critical analysis of the relationship between shoe-floor wear and pedestrian/walkway slip resistance. In: Marpet, M.

and Sapienza, M. editors. *Metrology of Pedestrian Locomotion and Slip Resistance*. American Society of Testing and Materials, Special Technical Publication 1424, ASTM International, Philadelphia. 33-48,

Kim, I.J., & Nagata, H. (2008a). Nature of the shoe wear: Its uniqueness, complexity and effects on slip resistance properties. *Contemporary Ergonomics 2008*, Taylor & Francis, 728-734.

Kim, I.J., & Nagata, H. (2008b). Research on slip resistance measurements - A new challenge. *Industrial Health*, *46*, 68-78.

Kim, I.J., Smith, R., & Nagata, H. (2001). Microscopic observations of the progressive wear on the shoe surfaces that affect the slip resistance characteristics. *International Journal of Industrial Ergonomics*, *28*, 17-29.

Kim, I.J., Hsiao, H., & Simeonov, P. (2013). Functional levels of floor surface roughness for the prevention of slips and falls: Clean-and-dry and soapsuds-covered wet surfaces. *Applied Ergonomics*, *44*, 58-64.

Leclercq, S., Tisserand, M., & Saulnier, H. (1993). Quantification of the slip resistance of metal surfaces at industrial sites. Part I. Implementation of a portable device, *Safety Science*, *17*, 29-39.

Ludema, K.C. (1987). Friction: a study in the prevention of seizure. *ASTM Standardization News*, *15(5)*, 54-58.

Manning, D.P., Jones, C., Rowland, F.J., & Roff, M. (1998). The surface roughness of a rubber soling material determines the coefficient of friction on water-lubricated surfaces. *Journal of Safety Research*, *29*, 275-283.

Menezes, P.L., Kailas, K., & Kailas, S.V. (2009). Study of Friction and Transfer Layer Formation in Copper-Steel Tribo-System: Role of Surface Texture and Roughness Parameters. *Tribology Transactions*, *52*, 611-622.

Miller, J.M. (1983). 'Slipper' work surfaces: towards a performance definition and quantitative coefficient of friction criteria. *Journal of Safety Research*, *14*, 145-158.

Moore, D.F. (1972). The friction and lubrication of elastomers, *International Series of Monographson Materials Science and Technology*, Pergamon Press Ltd., Headington Hill Hall, Oxford.

Moore, D.F. (1975). Principles and application of tribology, Pergamon Press, Oxford.

Murphy, T. (2003). Slip-resistant flooring. *The Society for Protective Coatings*. 390-396.

Proctor, T.D., & Coleman, V. (1988). Slipping and tripping accidents and falling accidents in Great Britain - present and future. *Journal of Occupational Accidents*, *9*, 269-285.

Rowland, F.J., Jones, C., & Manning, D.P. (1996). Surface roughness of footwear soling materials: relevance to slip-resistance. *Journal of Testing and Evaluation*, *24*, 368-376.

Scott, W.E. (2009). Falls at Work: Protect Your Employees: Statistics of Accidents, The National Safety Council.

Wilson, M.P. (1996). Slip resistance characteristics of footwear solings assessed using the SATRA friction tester. *Journal of Testing and Evaluation*, *24*, 377-385.

World Health Organization (WHO). (2007). WHO Global Report on Falls Prevention in Older Age. Available from: http://www.who.int/ageing/publications/Falls_prevention7March.pdf?ua=1.

Yeoh, H.T., Lockhart, T.E., & Wu, X. (2013). Non-fatal occupational falls on the same level. *Ergonomics*, *56*, 153-165.

Yoon, H.Y., & Lockhart, T.E. (2006). Nonfatal occupational injuries associated with slips and falls in the United States. *International Journal of Industrial Ergonomics*, *36(1)*, 83-92.

Yu, L., & Bahadur, S. (1998). An investigation of the transfer film characteristics and the tribological behavior of polyphenylene sulfide composites in sliding against tool steel. *Wear*, *214*, 245-251.

Zhao, Q., & Bahadur, S. (1998). A study of the modification of the friction and wear behavior of polyphenylene sulfide by particulate Ag2S and PbTe fillers. *Wear*, *217*, 62-72.

Zhao, Q., & Bahadur, S. (1999). The mechanism of filler action and the criterion of filler selection for reducing wear. *Wear*, *225-229*, 660-668.

INDEX

C

D

E

F

G

H

I

J

K

L

M

Q

R

S

T

U